I0487458

Cancer and You

Cancer and You

The Good News You Should Know

Joyce Trout

Copyright © 2008 by Joyce Trout.

ISBN: Softcover   978-1-4363-7722-5

All rights reserved. No part of this book may be reproduced or transmitted in any form or by any means, electronic or mechanical, including photocopying, recording, or by any information storage and retrieval system, without permission in writing from the copyright owner.

This book was printed in the United States of America.

To order additional copies of this book, contact:
Xlibris Corporation
1-888-795-4274
www.Xlibris.com
Orders@Xlibris.com
54290

TABLE OF CONTENTS

DISCLAIMER

THIS BOOKLET IS FOR INFORMATION ONLY. IT IS NOT TO TAKE THE PLACE OF COMPETENT MEDICAL CARE.

Find a natural healing doctor or a doctor who will monitor you and reduce the medication slowly as you improve your health by cutting out high fat and processed foods, sweets, etc. Do all of this under the supervision of your doctor. Check at your health food store for the address of a natural healing doctor near you. Herbal or other natural healing methods are not without possible allergic reactions.

All Services & Reports offered by Joyce Trout of Overton County are Religious in Nature & Not the Practices of Any Secular Scientific Healing Art.

Follow God's plan and He will bless.

Isaiah 63:9, "In all your afflictions He was afflicted" and 3 John 1:2 "Beloved, I wish above all things that thou mayest prosper and be in health, even as thy soul prospereth."

Some people have arrested chronic, degenerative disease by a total raw foods diet with live vegetable juices with an excellent detoxification program.

"Bless the Lord, O my soul, and forget not all his benefits: who forgiveth all thine iniquities; who healeth all thy diseases." Psalm 103:2-3.

The author dedicates this booklet to those who have undergone natural healing treatments to restore themselves to health.

INTRODUCTION

Thomas Edison once said, "The doctor of the future will give no medicine but will interest his patients in the care of the human frame in diet and in the cause and prevention of disease."

There are some positive steps known and practiced by a small group of researchers, medical doctors, and herbalists to prevent cancer and/or help to stop cancer growth and destroy tumors.

I have composed this study after over 40 years of research on herbs and natural healing methods. As time went by and information accumulated concerning these much-maligned subjects of herbs, healthy lifestyle, and God's natural laws, the dreaded disease of cancer came into view. I will show most people who are destined to die from cancer, do not have to die.

Americans are unhealthy considering how abundant is the supply of food and knowledge concerning exercise and proper eating habits. For instance, as of October, 1993, one out of eight American women will contract breast cancer. Every 12 minutes, a woman will die of breast cancer. According to 1990 statistics, one out of two Americans will contract cancer in their lifetime. It is in epidemic proportions.

I chose to speak out, as have many others, with deep concern over the state of medicine as we know it today. There is overwhelming evidence that our lifestyles of fast-food hamburgers, pizzas, continued consumption of meat, processed foods, refined sugar, refined white flour, and many, many other foods which are lined up on shelf after shelf in our supermarkets-continue to take its toll on the lives of our children, the elderly, yes, every one of us.

There is also overwhelming evidence that medical doctors are more adept at treating symptoms as opposed to the root causes of disease. Admittedly they are good at micro-surgery, orthopaedics, etc. but they fail to understand the need to treat the whole body—not just the symptom of the present disease.

God has left us the plans for the regeneration of the body if we will take the time to learn how to use the aids He has given us. In the very first chapter of Genesis, the Bible records that God made the herbs on the third day of creation. Then in the same first chapter, verse 29, "And God said, 'Behold I have given you every herb bearing seed which is upon the face of the earth; . . . to you it shall be for meat" and then God repeats, "I have given every green herb for meat" in verse 30.

Hippocrates, the Father of Medicine, used 29 herbs to cure every disease on the Island of Cos in the Greek Archipelago. In 400 B.C Hippocrates said that disease was a mysterious incident occurring in a mysterious universe, but that if the laws of the universe were adhered to, the body had the power to eliminate the disease. He believed that disease symptoms were a signal of movement toward health. The Hippocratic followers believed that they could not properly deal with disease by dealing with isolated symptoms one at a time, but only by working with all aspects of the patient simultaneously. He believed in the vital force God gave us.

Doctors argue that herbs are unproven remedies-unproven according to the medical profession in this country, but there are numerous case histories of people who have declined modern medicine and techniques and gone strictly with natural healing methods and have been successful in regaining health. (See "Case Histories" Section)

"People need to be taught that drugs do not cure disease. It is true that they sometimes afford present relief and the patient appears to recover as the result of their use. This is because nature has sufficient vital force to expel the poison and to correct the conditions that caused the disease. Health is recovered in spite of the drug. But in most cases, the drug only changes the form and location of the disease. Often the effect of the poison seems to be overcome for a time, but the results remain in the system and work great harm at some later time."[1]

---

[1]   E. G. White MH p. 126

WHAT IS CANCER?

There are three causes of any disease: (1)dehydration of the body (2) Too many poisons in the body & (3) acidosis or a very acidic body. This is also true of cancer, although the nature of cancer is multi-faceted. Dr. Ernest Wynder, President of American Health foundation said: "Dietary deficiencies lead to malfunctions of the body that cause cancer."

There are so many cases of cancer today because we have transgressed the health laws of God which God has told us about in Genesis and throughout the Bible. Cancer is the failure of the body to digest protein. A weakened immune system turns a healthy cell into a cancer cell. Cancer patients can get protein starved because the body is not digesting protein properly. If this condition continues, the body eats itself by attacking muscles to get protein which is why a person needs vegetable protein to rebuild the body.[2] If you crave sweets and starches, you are not getting enough vegetable protein. Stress further depletes the body of protein. Cancer is a stress related disease. Put yourself in the hands of the Great Physician. When you do your endorphin level goes up and you form B & T cells which help fight the cancer.

Fats rob the oxygen from the red blood cells. There is undissolved fat in the cancer cells. The body cannot digest fatty acids. Fats are deposited on arteries. This is because the liver and pancreas are sick. Diabetes is a fat metabolism problem, so is cancer. If we get too much sugar in the blood stream, the pancreas tries to produce insulin to counteract it. If this happens on a regular basis, the pancreas burns out trying to keep up with its insulin production. As the fats rob oxygen from the red blood cells, the walls collapse and we have high blood pressure and high cholesterol besides cancer or diabetes.

---

[2]   Protein needs are discussed in "The Lymphatic System."

When you have cancer, the pancreas is not putting out enough pancreatic protein digesting enzymes to digest the excess protein that is in the system because the pancreas and liver are sick. The cancer cell has a protein coating on it which needs to be digested so the white blood cells can destroy the cancer cell. When this doesn't happen, the cancer cells multiply and grow because of the partially digested protein floating around in the blood stream feeding the cancer cells. Cancer is systemic so a person needs to cleanse the blood as well as the whole body.

Wherever there is a weakness, a tumor forms. Animal protein feeds cancer because the dairy products and meats are high in fats and high in protein. They form uric acid and other poisons. A high protein diet of meat and dairy products kill you while it gives you energy because the meat rots in the colon and many poisons are expelled. Cancer lives on poisons. The cancer cell is a fermentative cell. The uric acid causes many other health problems like arthritis, gout, etc. Our colons were not made to accommodate meat. Short colon animals are meat-eaters. Our colons are two-thirds too long. Ask any gorilla what he eats and he will tell you, "fruits and vegetables." Undigested proteins such as beans feed the cancer cell as well. That is why the digestion has to be taken care of with an all plant enzyme such as Digest.

Meats, dairy, sugar, and substitute meat from the health food store damage the liver and the kidneys, too. It depends on how strong the liver and kidneys are before you suffer disease because of the poisons produced from animal proteins or highly processed & seasoned with lots of salt-meat substitutes. All cancer patients have parasites which live on poisons and toxins. They reproduce and cause other problems in the body if they are not destroyed. Black walnut tincture destroys parasites[3]—take for six months to one year for best results.

TYPES OF CANCER

There are numerous types of cancer which can afflict all parts of the body. While they all have in common a similar cellular structure abnormality they differ in body locations and severity. Treatment may be localized as follows, for example:

Lymphoma Cancer: If you have lumps in the groin area, under the arms, or anywhere else you may use the following poultice on them. Use 2-3 Tablespoons of each herb. Put one cup of water on to boil, lower the heat to

---

[3]   Fresh garlic will do the same.

simmer. Add powdered flaxseed and slippery elm while stirring slowly. Then add powdered charcoal while stirring very slowly. Put this mixture on a white cloth as hot as you can comfortably stand it. Put the poultice on the lumps in one area at a time. Cover this with plastic to keep in the heat and tape it or wrap it securely. Leave this on all night. If you have many lumps don't do the whole body at the same time as it may release too many poisons too fast. Keep doing this until the lumps or swellings go down in size and disappear. This poultice is excellent anywhere you have swelling externally. If there is infection you may add powdered goldenseal. Use this poultice only once as it draws out infection.

Breast Cancer: Use the poultice as described above but when you wrap the breast leave the nipple exposed so it can drain. This is a very sensitive area so don't have it too warm. You can use Dr. John Christopher's Black Salve for drawing out cancers. Black Salve is for all types of cancers that need the drawing power, for warts, moles, old ulcers, tumors, boils, & hemorrhoids. You will find it is very soothing & healing with slippery elm for breast cancer. Black Salve has the phenomenal ability to draw out cancerous toxins in the form of tumors. A tumor is a mass of toxins that have formed together. Black Salve is excellent for hardened liver & scanty bile flow. One man had a carcinoma on the back of his hand, with Black Salve it was soon gone.

LIFE IS IN THE CELLS

LYMPHATIC SYSTEM

The most important function of the lymphatic system is to keep the blood proteins circulating. Excess protein saps energy from working muscles. With a knowledge of how the lymphatic system works we can understand how excess protein not only saps energy from a muscle but it will sap the energy from any organ or area in the body where it accumulates. The lymphatic system has hundreds of nodes spaced along the channels, which serve as filters. They remove impurities as an oil filter does in a car. They trap anything harmful, such as, dead red blood cells, chemicals, etc. These filters are so efficient that the lymph they finally deliver to the blood stream is clean. They can get overwhelmed by invading organisms. Cancer cells often start and grow in the lymphatic channels. Fats become a problem in our lymphatic system because they absorb them from the intestines and dribble them into the blood stream slowly. The lymphatic system produces antibodies which destroy invading bacteria, and they manufacture 1/6 of the infection fighting white cells. They rush this little army to the scene of infection. There isn't any other way except the lymphatics for excess proteins (which seep out of the blood capillaries into the areas around the cells) to return to the circulatory system.

Even though a lymph system acts like a modern sewage treatment facility, it is literally the tree of life inside the body, because when this system fails to function properly, excess blood proteins along with excess fluid and poisons build up in the body and pain, loss of energy, infections, and disease will take place.[4] Remember any mental, emotional upset or muscular activity puts cells

---

[4]   Dr. C. Samuel West-he was a lymphologist.

to work and active cells emit poisons that must be transported by the lymph system so that we do not have trapped protein.

Our lymphatic system has roots in the feet, its branch in the head, and the tree trunk is in the chest area where the thoracic duct is located. If the lymphatic system is not working well, we have disease and then it is critical that we reactivate the lymphatics and our immune system. The lymphatic vessels have one way check valves that keep fluids going in one direction. The best way to get rid of trapped protein is through deep breathing and exercise. One suggested method of exercise is use a mini trampoline on a daily basis. You can get one at Wal-mart for around $20-$30. Keep your toes on the trampoline and just bounce & deep breathe. Lift the heels off slightly. Do this twice blowing out your breath each time. Deep breathe & hold the third breath then blow out all the air. This moves the lymphatic system and gets it to dump its poisons. If you feel sick or dizzy after a few bounces-quit for now. This means you need this exercise, but since you are releasing poisons and toxins while you are bouncing, it may make you feel sick. Buildup slowly as you get used to it. Stay on the minitrampoline for longer periods each time until you can bounce for longer periods of time and not get tired or feel sick. It may take awhile to build up.

If you cannot stand on the minitrampoline and bounce by yourself-sit on it with your feet on the minitrampoline and have someone stand behind you and bounce and deep breathe as you do the deep breathing, also. This will reactivate your friend's and your lymphatic system. Breathe deeply-inhale, exhale, inhale, exhale, inhale. Hold the last inhalation, then exhale, exhale, exhale. This causes the lymph to shoot into the blood stream like a geyser. This activates the immune system. Do this while bouncing on the minitrampoline.

Some people ask, "Well, why don't I die when this blood protein gets trapped if blood proteins can collapse your circulatory system?" This does happen in some cases. Some people go into extreme shock and die or have severe injuries which can result in death. The protein gets trapped quickly throughout the body. Dr. C. Samuel West says, "Our blood proteins can collapse our circulatory system and cause death as in traumatic or surgical shock, severe burns and accidental injuries. If the blood proteins get trapped slowly, the body will adjust to live in a sick or diseased state."

What Dr. West is saying is, in extreme cases, the person can die. Usually, the blood protein gets trapped slowly and the body adapts to the sickly condition. The results: aches, pains, and a general feeling of discomfort. We may have a muscle spasm, headache, loss of energy, or whatever. Oxygen plus glucose makes the lymphatic system work. Lack of oxygen, glucose and trapped blood proteins cause disease. Fruits, vegetables, and sprouts (complex carbohydrates) are the primary source of glucose. The brain needs a lot of glucose. People who are hypoglycemic need glucose constantly. Lack of glucose causes fainting.

Dr. Arthur C. Guyton says, "Complex carbohydrates in fruits, vegetables, and sprouts prevent weakness and reduce your need for protein." He goes on to say that carbohydrates are burned in preference to the burning of protein for energy, which is very important for preserving functional proteins in the cells.

A baby subsists on mother's milk and doubles and triples in size rapidly. The mother's milk is 2.38% protein at birth. This builds body cells. Funny, but you get the same percentage of protein in a baked potato, or carrot juice, or green leafy vegetables, the same amount the baby gets. Adults don't need as much protein as babies because we aren't building muscle, and tissue, etc as babies are doing. Just enough protein to maintain our body's needs daily. Vegetable proteins build body cells.

According to Dr. West "The more you eat right, the better you will feel, and the better you feel, the better you can eat right."

Our body cells are electrical. Each cell has an electric spark, which is the energy that the cells produce. Dr. Guyton, the leading lymphologist, stated in the Textbook of Medical Physiology, that our body must be in a "dry state" so the cells get oxygen and nutrients from the blood stream. There must be no trapped protein and no excess fluid around the cells, only enough fluid to fill the crevices around the cells. The live vital enzymes from raw vegetables, fruits, and fresh vegetable juices give the cells the electric spark similar to a spark plug in a car.

Each cell has potassium in it. Potassium is an enzyme catalyst or enhancer. When potassium is lost from the cellular system, the immune system and the whole enzyme system refuse to function. The blood serum can show high potassium in it. This means that the potassium has leaked out of the cells and is in the blood serum where it doesn't belong. Sodium rushes into the cells and fills the void. This imbalance inside the cell damages or kills them and causes every crippling or killer disease known to man. Sodium belongs in the blood serum and not in the cells. There is an energy exchange between the cells. When the chemical balance is right, the cells have the oxygen and nutrients they need to reproduce. Dr. West said, "Loss of energy, pain, disease and death begin at the cellular level. To promote healing, you need to breathe deeply, everywhere you go as often as possible."

Flood the cells with fresh vegetable juices, barley green juice, green drink and herbs. These are all high in potassium. A good combination of vegetable juices is carrot, spinach, lettuce, celery, and a little beet. Use the leaves of the turnips as they are very rich in calcium if you need extra calcium If you don't have all of these vegetables use carrot and spinach only or some other with them.

Animal and dairy products trap protein. The body manufactures cholesterol; when you take excess cholesterol into the body, cholesterol epoxides and other poisons are formed. The high cholesterol foods, animal and dairy products, are poison to the body.

"Cholesterol epoxides and other substances form from cholesterol of dairy products and animal products which cause cells to mutate, which will cause cancer. Research states that cholesterol levels correlate with a high rate of coronary heart disease, also. Salt, simple sugars, high fat and high cholesterol foods are the causes of all killer and crippling diseases such as heart attacks, strokes, cancer and obesity."[5]

Do not go on a fast if you have cancer or some other degenerative disease. Your body is already very depleted of live foods rich in potassium. Dr. Max Gerson said, "Healing means restoring all body functions to normal activity on their own. It doesn't mean cutting out a body part, burning, or poisoning with drugs. It means correcting the underlying problem so that all body functions can go back to normal. In every person there is a healing mechanism."

You must remember cancer or chronic disease is a total breakdown of the system. You must detoxify the system and reactivate the healing mechanism God has put in our bodies. All diseases are a breakdown of the liver. If your liver works well you are healthy.

THE MEDICAL PROFESSION AND CANCER

The United States is the sickest nation on earth. The medical profession and the huge cartel of cancer research associations continue to be unsuccessful in finding a cure for cancer. Chemotherapy, radiation and surgery are the only answers the medical profession has and it is a well-known fact that none of the above cures cancer. Chemotherapy is a form of mustard gas which was used during the Vietnam War. The medical profession has the theory that if you use small amounts of mustard gas it will destroy cancer. Rather, chemotherapy or radiation destroy the good cells in the body and further destroy the liver.

---

5   "Scientific American" Feb. 1977 issue

The tumor is not the cancer, it is just a symptom of a polluted toxic body. Chemotherapy destroys the white blood cells which fight infection.

Now let's take the American death ceremony. The death ceremony started as a crude ritual in the days of witchcraft. In recent years it has been developed into a science. It usually takes from 10-15 years; however, modern scientific advancements are shortening this period of time. It starts with one simple aspirin for a simple headache. When the one aspirin will no longer cover up the headache, you take two aspirins. After a few months when two aspirins will no longer cover up the headache, you take one of the stronger compounds. By this time it becomes necessary to take something for the ulcer that has been caused by the aspirin. Now you are taking two medicines. You have a good start.

After a few months, these medications will disrupt your liver functions. If a good infection develops you can take some penicillin. Of course, the penicillin will damage your red blood corpuscles and spleen so that you may develop anemia. Now another medication is then taken to cover up the anemia. And by this time, all these medications will put such a strain on your kidneys that they will break down. Now it's time to take some antibiotics. When these destroy your natural resistance to disease you can expect a general flare-up of all of your symptoms. The next step is to cover up all these symptoms with sulfa drugs. When the kidneys finally plug up, you can have them drained. Some poisons will build up in your system but you can keep going quite awhile this way by using the medications. By now, the medications will be so confused they won't know what they are supposed to be doing but it doesn't really matter. The body is thoroughly confused by now as to what the drugs are doing.

Dr. S. Weir Mitchell once said, "Back of disease lies a cause, and that cause no drug can reach." When a doctor diagnoses and tells his patients that they have three months to live, many of those patients choose to believe the doctor. Most will accept the verdict, for example, if the doctor says that the patient has diabetes and he'll "just have to live with it," or he'll be on insulin for the rest of his life. It'll just get worse." This causes the endorphin level to go down. The endorphins are the chemical messengers in the brain. They have natural morphine-like properties which suppress pain. Proverbs 17:22 says "A merry heart doeth good like a medicine but a broken spirit drieth the bones." Someone else comes along and says God's Plan will work for you. God can heal you if you eat fruits, vegetables, whole grains, seeds, and nuts and drink lots of raw vegetable juices and detoxify with herbs. Now the endorphin level goes up and the person begins to get well. Now there is hope.

How does chemotherapy act on healthy cells? "Unfortunately any cancer drugs can affect normal rapidly dividing cells, as well as cancer cells. Normal cells that might be affected include those in the bone marrow, gastrointestinal tract, reproductive system and the hair follicles."[6]

"And the light of a candle shall shine no more at all in thee; and the sound of a millstone shall be heard no more at all in thee . . . For thy merchants were the great men of the earth; for by thy sorceries were all nations deceived. And in her was found the blood of prophets and of saints, and of all that were slain upon the earth."[7]

"For by thy sorceries were all nations deceived," if traced back to the Greek, "sorceries" means "pharmacopoeia" or drugs. Now we have license to dispense legal drugs.

"Special instruction should be given in the art of treating the sick without the use of poisonous drugs and in harmony with the light God has given. In the treatment of the sick, poisonous drugs need not be used."[8]

"Multitudes remain in inexcusable ignorance in regard to the laws of their being. They are wondering why our race is so feeble, and why so many die prematurely. Is there not a cause? Physicians who profess to understand the human organism prescribe for their patients, even for their own dear children, and their companions, slow poisons to break up the disease or to cure slight indispositions. Surely, they cannot realize the evil of these things as they are presented to me or they could not do thus. The effects of the poison may not be immediately perceived, but it is doing its work undermining the constitution and crippling nature in her efforts. They are seeking to correct an evil but produce a far greater one which is often incurable."[9]

"Drugs always have a tendency to break down and destroy vital forces and nature becomes so crippled in her efforts that the invalid dies, not because she needed to die, but because nature was outraged. If she had been left alone she would have put forth her highest efforts to save life and health."[10]

The answer, my friends, is God's way the simple natural method of healing. "The true method of healing the sick is to tell them of the herbs . . . This is True Science."[11]

---

[6]   Chemotherapy & You pamphlet NIH p. 3

[7]   Rev. 18:23-24

[8]   Testimonies vol. 9 page 175

[9]   Spiritual Gifts vol. 4A 1864 page 137

[10]   Medical Ministry page 223

[11]   Ms. 105 1898

HOW TO PREVENT AND TREAT CANCER

First and foremost if you are serious about dealing with cancer, you must be willing to change your eating habits & your lifestyle. For example, get proper rest and exercise. Do deep breathing exercises every day, inhaling through your nose and exhaling through your mouth. Make up your mind that you will not eat between meals. Give up all meat and dairy products. Stop drinking soft drinks; stop eating refined foods and white sugar. You must forever forget about greasy hamburger, fried chicken, pizza, virtually all fast food restaurants. We must discipline that sweet tooth that draws us to the bakeries with the sugary pies, cakes, and brownies.

Getting back to God's simple menu of fresh fruits, fresh vegetables, nuts, whole grains, seeds, and plenty of good water is the big step each one of us must be willing to take. Now you are feeding the body the live vital enzymes which are needed for our whole body metabolism. Ask the Lord to take away the desire for foods that don't nourish and strengthen the body and He is faithful to fulfill your wish for good health.

VITAMINS

Vitamin A: This protects us from infections. It aids in the growth and repair of body tissue. It puts oxygen in the blood; it is a fat soluble vitamin. It can be stored in the body. There is no danger of getting too much in fresh raw foods. Carrot juice is your best source of Vitamin A. Make it fresh every day. One carrot has 11,000 I.U.'s of Vitamin A in its juice.

Vitamin A helps eyesight, builds strong bones and teeth and maintains rich blood. Recent research has found that Vitamin A can enhance the body's defense against invaders as common as respiratory infections and as deadly as cancer. Vitamin A in an emulsified form has been used in conjunction with laetrile in biological treatment of cancer in Germany, the country that leads the world in cancer weapons that destroy cancer naturally. It helps maintain alkalinity in the body. It protects the body from kidney stones & gall stones. All these show a deficiency of Vitamin A.

Vitamin B6 may be an important link in the treatment and prevention of cancer. It helps by hunting down and destroying malignant cells. White blood cells need B6 to manufacture antibodies. It is needed for white blood cells or lymphocytes to hunt and destroy cancer. B6 foods: High fiber whole grains, fruits, vegetables, potatoes, tomatoes, whole wheat, wheat germ, garlic, black strap molasses, nuts, and all types of seeds.

Vitamin B12 gives the body an acid bath to allow iron to be absorbed. Comfrey and alfalfa are two plants that contain Vitamin B12. You may make them as tea.

Vitamin B17: Eat green vegetables, lentil sprouts, mung bean sprouts, garbanzos, buckwheat, millet, flaxseed, apple seeds, lima beans, pears, plums, peaches, cherry seeds, prunes, lettuce, kidney beans, corn and almonds. The pits of all the fruit contain Laetrile or B17 so eat them.

Vitamin C Strengthens the lymphocytes which fight viral infections. It has interferon in it which fights different viruses. It will prevent or cure the common cold. It contributes to the health of the arteries and is helpful to the circulatory system. It can prevent advancing age. Every part of the body benefits from Vitamin C. If you are susceptible to infections, you may need more foods rich in Vitamin C. For example: strawberries, green peppers, citrus fruits, broccoli, brussel sprouts, cabbage, guavas, kale, mustard greens, turnip greens, tomatoes, fresh peas, cauliflower, kohlrabies, and watercress.

Vitamin E an antioxidant protects the heart along with the Edenic diet of fruits, vegetables, whole grains, seeds, and nuts (sunflower seeds are the richest source of Vitamin E), toasted wheat germ, filberts, almond and pine nuts.

Antioxidants are radical scavengers which hunt down and neutralize oxygen free radicals in the cell system in seconds. Antioxidants put oxygen into the blood. Vitamins E, A, and C, B-6, selenium, zinc rich foods such as pumpkin seeds and garlic contain antioxidants, walking every day and deep breathing oxygenate the system and destroy toxins. Cancer can't live in an oxygen rich environment. Strokes, heart attacks, cancer, etc occur because of free radical damage to the cells but this cell damage can be reversed. Scientists compared the ability of old and young gerbils when they ran a complex maze. The older gerbils made 2.5 times as many mistakes as the young. When the older gerbils were given a powerful antioxidant they were able to run the maze almost as fast as the young gerbils. The older gerbils have lower levels of brain chemicals or neurotransmitters. Their brain cells have been damaged by free radicals. Free radicals are the cause of oxidation in our tissues, their proliferation is favored by stress, poor diets, and the pollution of the environment. When they take antioxidants, the neurotransmitter levels rise markedly and the damaged brain cells return almost to normal. Raw vegetable juices taken during the day between your meals at the rate of 2 quarts a day will put lots of antioxidants into your system. Cells thus protected quickly regain their regenerative power.

Stimulators are brain foods which give the brain more oxygen and nourish it like gingko, kotu kola, Vitamin E, & niacin.

If you have had any chemotherapy or radiation in order to counteract it take barley green often during the day. It may be taken every hour or two. I would take the green drink, also, as stated in this paper as this rebuilds the immune system and counteracts the effects of the radiation and chemotherapy.

MINERALS

Potassium: The beginning of all chronic disease is loss from the cells of potassium and sodium rushes into the cells but it doesn't belong in the cells. The building of almost all enzymes in the body requires potassium as a catalyst and is inhibited by sodium. So, in order to initiate the healing, it is essential to remove the excess sodium from the cells and reintroduce large amounts of potassium. This is best made from fresh carrots, apple, and green vegetable juices. Drink at least 2 quarts a day. Fruit is rich in potassium, it helps control blood pressure. The fruit washes sodium out of the cells and rebuilds the immune system. This detoxifies the system of accumulated toxins. Potassium acts as an activating substance within each cell. Cancerous cells can't live in potassium.

Calcium: if it is organic, is an enzyme activator. Its effects are important in fighting viral infections. The more organic calcium and magnesium we have in our diets, the less chance of heart disease since organic calcium lowers serum cholesterol. Calcium is depleted when one is under stress as with some major disease, etc. When we have a virus, for example, the body needs lots of organic calcium as in carrot juice. Green leafy vegetables, nuts, & seeds are rich in calcium. Carrot juice is rich in calcium as well as many other vitamins & minerals.

Magnesium is the regulator of minerals. Use magnesium rich foods such as all the seeds, barley, almonds, lima beans, corn, oatmeal, peas, brown rice, whole grains, whole wheat flour, hazel nuts, Brazil nuts, cashews, pecans, & soy flour. Chelated magnesium protects the heart. Young athletes who suddenly died of a heart attack with no prior heart problems were low in magnesium. Chelated magnesium is a good insurance against heart attacks. Chelating foods: onions, garlic, cayenne, chives, asparagus, peas, lima beans, pintos, kidney beans, soybeans, & other legumes, sesame seeds, pumpkin seeds, sunflower seeds, and walnuts.

Zinc nourishes the thymus gland and builds lymphocytes to fight viral infections. Pumpkin seeds are rich in zinc. A lack of zinc interferes with the formation of the nucleus of the cell. Zinc is found in all human tissues. It is essential for the synthesis of body protein and the action of many enzymes.

Iron: The body does not use iron properly if we have cancer so you can become anemic. The following are some iron rich foods: black strap molasses, red beets, grape juice, watermelon, strawberries, raisins, apricots, tomatoes, asparagus, figs, celery, parsley, prunes, wheat germ. Eat a lot of raw foods. Iron carries oxygen in the blood and cancer cannot live where there is oxygen. Do not take iron tablets or liquid iron as they are not used properly; get your iron from iron rich foods in the organic state which is raw. I have an iron drink recipe that is excellent.

Selenium destroys free radicals or the cancer cells. Selenium is an antioxidant. It boosts the immune system and preserves young vital cells by helping to block cellular aging initiated by oxidation. The incidence of breast cancer was reduced from 82 % to 10% when 2 parts per million was added to the drinking water of experimental mice, according to G. N.
Schrauzer and D. Ann Ismael. A rule of thumb is that the average person needs 200 mcg. of selenium each day. Selenium sources include bread made from fresh ground winter wheat, bee pollen, Brazil nuts (4 nuts equal 210 mcg), & raw coconut (one ounce equals 225 mcg).

Iodine for the healthy function of the thyroid is found in spinach, loose-leaf lettuce, carrots, beans, peas, turnips, cabbage, tomatoes, onions, radishes, & watercress to name a few. Parsley & white oak bark tea aid in normal function of the thyroid.

VEGETABLE PROTEINS

You need vegetable protein because these are the building blocks of the body. Our bodies are made of protein. The vegetable protein builds and repairs the body. Vegetable protein builds new cells, tissue, organs, skin, hair, nails, and even our bones are made of protein. We only need 25-30 grams of protein a day. Meat & dairy protein when it is heated to 150 degrees becomes denatured undigestible protein that the body can't use. Americans that eat meat & dairy get 90-100 grams of protein a day & this high protein diet takes calcium out of the body. That is why we have so much osteoporosis in the USA. This protein feeds the cancer cell big time, also. God created us to be vegetarians. The animals eat the meat raw so they get the proteins they need plus they have a short colon so it goes thru quickly. We have 26 feet of colon so the meat protein stays in our colon 2-3 days & rots. The only protein that the body uses is the vegetable protein. You can get this protein from green leafy vegetables, sesame seeds-ground, sunflower seeds-ground or eaten raw, soybeans, wheat germ, nuts, peas, lentils, whole wheat grains, potatoes, barley, vegetable juices, much more. Bee pollen is a good source of vegetable protein and it gives you energy. Tofu contains a large amount of protein but it isn't good for a cancer patient as it contains too much protein. Eat it once a week after you get well. I have a paper on High Protein diet if you want it.

HERBS

Herbs are electrical just as our bodies are electrical. The herbs put energy back into the cells and potassium. Herbs stimulate the white blood corpuscles which absorb and destroy germs. Herbs regulate organs and glands and correct imbalance. Herbs cleanse each cell. Herbs and diet work hand in hand. Herbs feed the body the vitamins and minerals and are rich in potassium. The body needs to work in the proper balance and ratio that God intended. Herbs work with nature in the healing process. They can rebuild and detoxify the body if you use them correctly.

Comfrey (knitbone)-heals wounds and ulcers even if down to the bone. The allantoin is a cell proliferant and healing agent, stimulating healthy tissue growth. Comfrey is high in potassium, vegetable protein, and calcium. Comfrey regenerates the brain, nerve tissue, and bones. It heals whatever it comes in contact with such as broken bones, pulled muscles, etc. It is good for delicate digestive organs. You can stop hemorrhage with a tea made from comfrey powder because it is mucilaginous & soothing to the whole body.

Dandelion contains more Vitamin C than tomatoes and 20% more Vitamin A than carrots. Dandelion is rich in calcium, iron, potassium, sulfur and many other minerals. It is a liver and blood cleanser, relieves ulcers, stomach disorders, joint and muscle stiffness. The leaves & the root of the dandelion plant combined with carrot & turnip leaves juice assists in remedying spinal and bone problems as well as it gives strength and firmness to the teeth.

Chickweed: This tea soothes and heals whatever it comes in contact with such as congestion of the liver. It is excellent for all types of chest problems like pleurisy, bronchitis, any kidney problems, rheumatism and the stomach. It is good for ulcerated throat and mouth, swellings, boils, and blood poisoning. It dissolves fats and tumors. Chickweed is rich in potassium, iron, and calcium.

Mullein: Use mullein for the lungs and all internal irritations. It rids the body of mucus. It is excellent for asthma, hay fever, allergies, sinus, nervous disorders, heart conditions, shortness of breath, and all lung problems. It is used for childhood epilepsy and headaches. Great for hemorrhage of the colon. You take 1 oz. of powdered mullein and heat 1 pint of whole cow's milk. Stir the mullein into the hot tea. Drink this after each bowel movement. The reason for the milk is that it has so much casein in it that the milk glues the mullein on the walls of the intestinal tract and stops the bleeding. The only good use for milk is for glue. It works great.

Juniper berry: It builds immunity. It is a good digest aid. You need a good digest aid when you have cancer because the body isn't breaking down the fats & the proteins so the undigestible protein is feeding the cancer cell. The pancreas isn't producing the digestive enzymes because it is sick and it doesn't have enough of the pancreatic enzymes. You have a very acidic condition so you need to make it more alkaline by eating raw foods and drinking raw vegetable juices. Juniper berry tea is good for the kidneys. It is a diuretic. Don't take if the kidneys are inflamed or weak.

Black Walnut Tincture reduces lymphatic swelling. It disables and disintegrates parasites. You need to take it for 6 months to one year to rid the body of unwanted "guests". It contains iodine for the thyroid.

Bayberry (bardana) is high in copper. Copper attaches itself to and removes excess deposits of inorganic calcium in the body. This relieves congestion of the lymphatics. Bayberry is a wonderful herb for the sinus. You make a tea and snuff it up the nostrils.

Chaparral cleans the blood. It is effective for the following: prostate trouble, skin and stomach cancer, leukemia, arthritis, warts, bronchitis, & much more. It is antifungal, antibacterial, and antibiotic.

Sheep or wood sorrel (for skin cancer): Put the herb through the juicer. Let the bowl of juice evaporate so it gets thick or gelatinous in the bowl. Apply to the skin cancer for a week or more, apply several times a day. It will pull out the roots of the cancer and leave a little hole. Put hydrogen peroxide and olive oil on the area. It will heal in a week or two. If you do not want the cancer to return follow the program in my Cancer book.

Green Drink: This acts as a blood transfusion to the body. Start with the best water in the blender. Throw in fresh picked dandelion, chickweed, plantain, parsley, lettuce, comfrey or spinach. If you don't have all of them throw in whatever green leaves you have. Blend well and strain. Drink as much as you can. It gives you energy & boosts the immune system.

Garlic and Horseradish combination is excellent for all kinds of problems in the body. It cleans out mucus and cleans the blood stream. Garlic helps to prevent the arteries from clogging and it dissolves the cholesterol. Garlic slows down the build up of fatty deposits on artery walls. It destroys any infectious germs in the body. The Horseradish is a stimulant, diuretic, antiscorbutic, antiseptic, germicide, vermicide, powerful digestant, and an expectorant. It is used in dropsy, paralysis, indigestion, rheumatism, dyspepsia, sciatica, poor circulation, malnutrition, pulmonary complaints, bronchitis, sinus problems, cancer & other diseases, & low blood pressure.

Dr. Maude Scott has a powerful formula she shares with us. Mix 2 & ½ bulbs of garlic and ½ inch of horseradish in the blender with one pint of the best water. Liquefy the garlic & horseradish by blending well. Add one more pint of water. Take one fourth cup of the mixture, put in an 8 oz. glass and fill the rest of the way with tomato juice or apple juice. Take one tablespoon of the mixture three times a day or more. This warms you up from head to toe. Drink it slowly to let it diffuse throughout the body. If this is still too potent add more apple or tomato juice to it. It activates the salivary glands, activates the sinus, opens up the bronchial tubes, cleans the lung area, cleans plague out of the blood stream and much more. Mrs E. G. White said: "The herbs that grow for the benefit of man and the little handful of herbs kept and steeped and used for sudden ailments have served tenfold, yes, one hundred-fold better purposes than all the drugs hidden under mysterious names and dealt out to the sick."

Again she said: "The Lord has given some simple herbs of the field and if every family were educated in how to use these herbs in case of sickness, much suffering might be prevented, and no doctor need be called. These simple herbs, used intelligently, would have recovered many sick who have died under drug medication." (Letter 82, 1897)

CLEANSING COMBINATION TEA

We know the life of the person is in the blood. Dr. John Christopher considered the bloodstream so important he called it "The River of Life." All disease stems from the blood. Someone can have a bad case of boils. The doctor can lance them and drain the boils but this doesn't solve the internal problem which is a polluted bloodstream. You are only treating the symptom when you treat the boil and don't cleanse internally. We need to get to the cause to not have the boils come back again. The impurities and poisonous waste accumulations in a boil are brought to that point by a bloodstream loaded with waste. Cleansing the bloodstream gets to the cause of the problem which is lots of poisons.

This same thing applies to cysts, tumors, cancer, dermatitis, etc. The weakened or injured parts or organs accumulate toxins because the blood is too weak to discard the body's toxins and poisons. You can have the surgeon cut out the tumor but it will come back again unless you clean the bloodstream and feed the body the live enzymes with raw vegetable juices, diet, & etc. Dr. John Christopher said," If you have a clean bloodstream you have no more disease." Cancer is systemic, the tumor is just a localized manifestation of an internal problem. The tumor is an accumulation of poisons. It occurs when the wastes accumulate in one area that is weak. The surgeon can cut out the tumor and the person can still die because he is only treating the symptom.

LEV. 17:11 says "For the life of the flesh is in the blood." We need to cleanse the blood with alterative herbs which alter and correct impure conditions of the blood. There are many causes for impure blood, you may have an organ or organs of the body that aren't functioning properly. Sometimes the secretory organs fail to carry out the impurities from the blood. Improper food, impure air, toxic chemicals, not enough live enzymes, & stress all play a part in the destruction of our bodies. If we try to cleanse the bloodstream with Dr. John Christopher's Cleansing Combination tea and continue to eat meats, dairy, concentrated starches, sweets, harmful drinks such as coffee, caffeine sodas, etc. it will not do us any good because we are polluting the bloodstream as fast as the herbal teas are trying to cleanse it.

Cleansing Combination Tea slowly cleans and purifies the bloodstream and tones up the organs to help remove the impurities from the blood. Our largest eliminative organ is our skin. The tea eliminates the waste from the cells, too. The liver, kidneys, skin, lungs, and colon need to be working properly.

Dr. John Christopher & Chief Sundance received the Red Clover Combination Tea from the good Lord in answer to the needs of their people. It is God's Cancer formula. It contains herbs which work together to detoxify the liver, spleen, lymphatics, colon, pancreas, cells, and bloodstream, etc. It relieves congestion and stagnation in the lymphatic system. It has a mild laxative effect when you drink it. It cleanses the whole body as I may have missed an organ it cleanses.

You may drink the tea at the rate of 2-6 cups a day. See what fits you the best depending on your physical condition. You may use it as a compress on tumors, also. One man used it on a facial tumor and in two months it was gone. Start with a pot of boiling water and add more tea than normal so it is strong. The more concentrated the better for a compress. Turn off and let it steep for 4-6 hours covered. Slow cook it until you have half the amount of tea you started with and now it is very strong for external use only. Strain & dip a white cloth in the warm tea and apply to the skin cancer, etc. Put plastic over the compress to keep in the moisture. Keep it on all night.

Dr. Christopher had as a patient a woman with RH negative problems. All three of her children had RH negative problems. She wanted one more child but her physician warned her she would probably kill herself and her unborn child. Besides, she was further weakened from open heart surgery. This woman went to see Dr. Christopher for advice. He put her on Cleansing Combination Tea to purify her blood, & the mucusless diet.

Several years later while he was giving a lecture in Idaho, this woman whom he hadn't seen since prescribing the Cleansing Combination Tea introduced him to her baby. She told him the baby had perfectly normal blood. They didn't have to drain the baby's blood as they did with her other three children. She had a perfect delivery. A few years later she had two more perfectly healthy children with normal blood.

The Cleansing Combination Tea is excellent but we have pockets of old garbage in the intestines from years of eating sweets, meats, dairy products, greasy foods, canned and processed foods so we need to stay on the tea for as long as it takes to clean the blood which may be up to a year. We need the raw vegetable juices, fresh fruits, vegetables, whole grains, seeds, and nuts. Remember there is not one magic answer to disease it is a total lifestyle change. Unless we are willing to monitor what goes in the front door we can't have a healthy body.

PARSLEY ROOT TEA

Parsley Root Tea has a remarkable ability to expel flatulence, watery poisons, excess mucoid matter, reduce swollen, enlarged glands, cystitis, irritation and inflammation of the kidneys. Use 4 ounces of parsley root to 2 quarts of the best water. Boil slowly in a covered pan for twenty minutes. Strain through cloth. Give one half to one teacupful of hot tea every hour. Take one pint of this tea and add one pint of vegetable glycerine. USE THIS FOR A HOT FOMENTATION ONLY. Saturate white cloths in hot tea and apply to the edematous areas.

First apply to the lumbar region and then to other edematous areas for 30 minutes. Cover with plastic and a bath towel. Apply an electric pad at a comfortable temperature over this. Apply a cold towel not iced over the areas for one minute after the 30 minute fomentation is taken off. If you perform the procedure as outlined, there will soon be a free flow of urine, the pores of the skin will relax and open permitting profuse perspiration and thus relieving the kidneys. People close to death and given up as hopeless have been relieved and restored to perfect health. Don't let the person get chilled. Keep them well covered in bed with some ventilation in the room.[12]

COMBINED DIETARY REGIME

The treatment of a combined dietary regime requires guidance from a natural healing physician because there may be complications of "flare ups" and activation of chronic infections, or other bodily weaknesses which need special medical attention. This is an intensive program if the person has cancer.

Necessary Food: This diet is quite different from the usual nutrition. It consist mainly of fruit, juices of fruit, vegetables and leaves, vegetable juices,

---

[12]   Purchase vegetable glycerin at your local health food store. Always use *vegetable* glycerin. This is for external use only. Glycerin penetrates as a softening, soothing, and healing agent for irritated skin surfaces.

salads, special soup, potatoes, oatmeal, whole wheat bread, all freshly prepared and salt free. The dietary regime is the basis of the treatment. The main task is to detoxify the entire system and to restore the functions of the liver and the metabolism. You need help with the digestion such as Digest. The cancer patient needs to flood the cells with potassium and needs to rebuild the immune system quickly. Eat large portions of the fruits and vegetables. Drink lots of vegetable juices.

Forbidden Foods include those which are bottled, canned, frozen, preserved, refined, salted, smoked or processed. Forbidden are berries, commercial beverages, bicarbonate of soda found in foods, ice cream, fatty foods, white flour, mushrooms, candy, cake, chocolate, cocoa, perked or instant coffee of any kind, cream, butter even the soy butter, cheese, eggs, nuts except almonds-rich in B17 & eat the pits of the seeds, use only flaxseed oil, spices, white & refined sugar, tea containing caffeine (use herb tea only), fish, meat of all kinds, milk & all dairy products. After the cancer is under control stick to a good diet of fruits, vegetables, whole grains, seeds, & nuts so it doesn't come back.

Also forbidden are alcohol, hair dyeing and permanents, fluoride toothpaste, gargles, epsom salts, nicotine, salt & substitutes. Do not use pressure cookers or any aluminum pans or utensils.

Use only fresh fruits (no fruits in cans), eat in large quantities-apples, apricots, bananas, cherries, currants, grapes, grapefruit, mangoes, melons, oranges, peaches, pears, plums, etc. Stewed fruits may be used. Use only unsulphured dried fruits such as raisins, dates, figs, prunes, etc. You may wash, soak & stew them.

For some people berries and pineapples have aromatic acids that can cause unfavorable reactions. Taken from A Cancer Therapy by Dr. Max Gerson, MD p. 237-238.

The pectin in apples is good for the colon. The apples are rich in potassium & the richest in oxygen of any fruit. Do not peel the apples. Wash in lemon juice water or add a bit of Miracle 2 soap(all natural soap) to the water in a dishpan. Let the apples soak for awhile. Use as much organic as you can find. Look in Dr. N W Walker's Fresh Vegetable & Fruit Juice book to see which vegetable combination is best for you. Usually it is carrot, spinach, & red beet juice.

Use as many of the following as possible: Loose-leaf lettuce, red cabbage leaves, beet tops, Swiss chard, escarole, endive, romaine, green pepper, watercress. Drink at least 2 quarts of the vegetable juice every day but more

is better. This puts oxygen into the blood & disease can't live where there
is oxygen. It cleanses each cell & puts the potassium back into the cells &
rebuilds the immune system so the body can heal itself.

You should eat one meal per day with no protein so the body has a chance
to digest the protein coating on the cancer cells so they can be destroyed. If
you eat protein every meal the pancreas has to produce the protein digestive
enzymes to digest the protein foods before it can digest the protein coating
on the cancer cell. Maybe eat only fruit at night so the body can work on
destroying the cancer cells while you are asleep. This gives the digestive system
a rest as fruit digests in one half hour.

Dr. John Christopher has a paperback called Herbal Home Health Care
which is an excellent reference book. You might want to add it to your library.
It gives a lot of help on what to do for different health problems.

THE COLON

Over 90% of all diseases are the result of an unclean intestinal tract, constipation, retention of feces, and lack of coordination in the nerve and muscle functions of the colon and bowel. "Within the body we find a backed up sewage line (constipation). We have 26 feet of pipe (small and large intestine). The horrible odor of halitosis comes out of the front door (mouth) as it is opened."[13] It is like a bathroom which has a stopped up toilet. It runs over and you smell the horrible odor. You can take a breath mint or use mouth wash. This only covers up the problem. This is the body's way of saying, "You have a toxic bowel condition."5 Cleaning out the vehicle of man and getting a tuneup is the most important thing in life: having a smoothly operating body that will use less fuel (food) and get better mileage and performance with a smooth operation.

Remember digestion begins in the mouth. "Chew each mouthful thoroughly, whether juice or solid food. Mix it with saliva. Without saliva mixed thoroughly with food or juice, the material goes into the stomach and it is eliminated without proper assimilation. The average person utilizes about 10% of his food value and the rest is wasted on down the eliminative drain. With the intestinal tract so badly layered and clogged, your food simply cannot get through to the absorptive villi and functional tissues on the walls and the usual result is that the bowel weakens, loses its elasticity and balloons out."[14] These hardened layerings in the bowels are just like rings in a tree, which are added to during each year and body degeneration will continue.

---

[13] *Herbal Home Health Care*, by Dr. John R. Christopher, N.D., and published by Christopher Publications p 129.

[14] Ibid P. 133

One person asked, "Why is it that I only eat one-fifth of what I used to eat, and when I was eating five times as much I had a bowel movement every day and I thought that was adequate; but now I am eating only one-fifth of what I formerly ate, I am having five to seven bowel movements each and EVERY day—and they are MASSIVE ones, and I am eating LESS."[15] Now he has MORE strength, MORE endurance, MORE pep and energy than ever before and he is HAPPIER.

"You will be able to go 3-4 times as long on the same quantity of food. "Bodily activity is another way of mechanically stimulating the intestine. Vigorous exercise sets the diaphragm and abdominal muscles at work so the intestines are stimulated to action."

A common misnomer held by medical men is that the stool should be "formed". The vegetarian Hindus, who live chiefly on ground wheat and vegetables have "large, bulky, and not formed, but pultaceous stools."

"A well formed stool always means constipation. The significance is that the colon is packed full like a sausage and that the fecal matters have been so long retained that they have been compacted by the absorption of water. The whole colon is filled, and the bowel movement is the result of the pressure of incoming food residues at the other end. When the body wastes are promptly discharged as they should be, the colon never contains the residues of more than two meals and at the after-breakfast movement should be completely emptied so that the disinfecting and lubricating mucus which its walls secrete may have the opportunity to cleanse and disinfect the body's garbage receptacle and thus keep it in a sanitary condition."[16]

Our body is made up of 75-80 percent fluid and it must be replaced by liquids every day. "The use of inorganic drinks (soft drinks) and beverages high in sugar, synthetic, sweetenings, and artificial colorings, the use of alcoholic beverages and polluted tap waters is as ridiculous as pouring salt, sugar, or dirty water into the gas tank of your car."[17]

---

[15]   Ibid PP. 135-136
[16]   *ibid*, pp 138-139.
[17]   *ibid*, pp 147-148.

The Colon Defined

The colon is a portion of the large intestine, a tubular, alimentary canal about five feet in length and two-and-one-half inches in diameter. The colon, the largest single section of the large intestine and the area of discussion here, extends from the caecum to the rectum and includes the sigmoid fixture.[18] As food passes from the small intestine through the ileocecal valve, it fills the caecum and accumulates in the ascending colon. Movements of the colon begin when substances enter through the ileocecal valve. As the caecum and the ascending colon fill, there begins a peristaltic wave in the middle of the transverse colon which drives the colonic contents along to their final destination.

Since chyme[19] moves through the small intestine at a fairly constant rate, the time required for a meal to pass into the colon is determined by its gastric evacuation time. What Are The Colon's Functions?

The colon serves to finish the digestion process begun in the small intestine. The intestinal walls have cells which secrete mucus which lubricates the colonic contents as they pass through the colon. Bacteria work on the chyme which is prepared for elimination. Bacteria ferment any remaining carbohydrates and release hydrogen, carbon dioxide and methane. These gases convert remaining proteins into amino acids and break down the amino acids into simpler substances, some of which is carried off and can be detected by its distinctive odor. The rest is transported to the liver for conversion to less toxic compounds and excreted.

---

[18]   For comparison, a small intestine is divided into three segments. The duodenum, the shortest part, originates at the pyloric sphincter of the stomach and extends about 10 inches until it merges with the jejunum. The jejunum is about 8 feet long and extends to the ileum. The final portion of the small intestine, the ileum, measures about 12 feet and joins the large intestine at the ileocecal valve. See page 610 of *Principles of Anatomy and Physiology*, 4th Ed. Tortora and Anagnostakos.

[19]   Chyme is the semifluid mass of partly digested food.

STEPS TO TAKE FOR
A HEALTHY COLON

To keep the colon working well, take lower bowel capsules (such as Dr. Christopher's Fen LB, following the directions on the label).[20] The colon should work by morning. Drink 2 qts. of water or herb tea all day. The LB capsules act as a food to aid the colon in working more efficiently. Undigested food in the fecal matter is a sign that the bowel is badly clogged and the food is not being assimilated.

If the colon doesn't work by morning take 16 oz. of hot water with a fresh squeezed lemon. This stimulates the colon to work. It is rich in potassium. It nourishes the brain and nerves, too. It is rich in Vitamin C, dissolves uric acid, flushes the liver and gall bladder. If the colon isn't working well, your liver is loaded with saturated fats so keep working on flushing it with everything I've mentioned in this paper.

Here are additional steps you can take: Take 2 probiotic capsules before each meal, particularly if you have been or are now taking drugs prescribed by a doctor. Probiotic puts friendly bacteria in the colon which drugs destroy. We need the friendly bacteria to keep the peristaltic motion in the colon and to eat up the unfriendly bacteria.

Take brisk walks to stimulate the bowels, breathing deeply as you walk. Proper exercise is important for proper bowel activity. Eat fresh roughage every day such as raw vegetables.

---

[20]   If the recommended dosage fails to restore a natural elimination rhythm, you may need to increase the dosage. One patient is on record as having taken 40 capsules per day to achieve regularity.

Drink fresh vegetable juices to flush out and cleanse the blood stream and kidneys while putting vitamins, minerals, enzymes and potassium into the cell system, forcing out the sodium which is not supposed to be in the cells.

Don't eat between meals. Eat every five to six hours, two or three times a day. Eat a light meal at night, preferably fruit. If food is allowed to digest properly, the bowels function properly. Eat only whole grain cereals, such as, oat groats from the health food store. Grind up sunflower seeds, sesame seeds and sprinkle them on your cereals. They are rich in vitamins and vegetable protein. Find a good recipe for making your own whole grain cereals, if you wish.

Remember all disease starts in the colon. Dr Kellogg said in his 22,000 colon operations he never saw a healthy colon. I am including material for cleansing the colon. You can't help the body's organs if you don't cleanse the colon. It is like putting more garbage in a garbage pail that is already overflowing.

Cascara Sagrada is an excellent herb to stimulate the peristaltic motion in the colon. This is the plant animals in nature nibble on to stay regular. Cascara Sagrada gives the bowel the strength to move. Responsible people enjoy the benefit of this herb to obtain one easy and complete bowel movement per meal just as was intended by nature. Bowel wastes removed more frequently in this way prevent all manner of mischief including prostate and uterus problems, bladder and urinary disorders, the hysterectomy, ear, throat, lung, liver, eye, sinus, and infections, etc. Bowel wastes when not frequently eliminated are reabsorbed from the colon into the rest of the body and they seek to be eliminated through emergency exits as skin, lungs, ears, throat, sinuses, etc.

Dr. A. B. Howard once said that "if you made Cascara Sagrada a habit, it became a good habit. The body no longer has to try and deal with backed-up bowel poisons and a new day dawns." Energy surges back into the body as a side effect of good bowel management.

You may want to use an enema once in a while with a mild tea as catnip or lemon juice water but do not use on a regular basis as this instills a dependency which forestalls natural elimination. In other words, no enema, no movement.[21]

---

[21] For the chronically ill or dying patient I would use only Cascara Sagrada capsules for detoxification.

PROLAPSED COLON

Psalms 104:14 "He causeth the grass to grow for the cattle, and the herb for the service of man; that he may bring forth food out of the earth." We wouldn't be here today if it wasn't for the herbs. The herbs are every growing thing that stays in one place. They contain phytonutrients.

We need to use all the herbs in their wholesome state. This allows life to generate with great strength. When we break down the foods we lose a lot of their value, for example the wheat. You extract the bran, heart, and the oil. We have a pretty white flour left that is good for nothing. It can't sustain life—even the bugs don't want it! The white flour is lifeless, it is worthless. It can't build a strong body. We are getting a weaker and weaker race. We need to eat foods in their wholesome state-fruits, vegetables, whole grains, seeds, and nuts. This will give your body the vitamins and minerals it needs that can be assimilated. Don't rush down to the health food store and get Vitamin A, B1, B3, etc. These aren't in their wholesome state as in fresh foods. Many "foods" that are highly advertised are not foods but only fillers that are loaded with mucus and they glue themselves on the side walls of the bowel. The closer they get to the outside the harder they get until we have a mucus casing around the wall of the bowel itself that is as hard as a plastic pipe. It has taken years to get in this condition. Now the food can't be assimilated through this casing. You may be assimilating 7-10% of your food if you are lucky. We need to get rid of this mucus lining so we can assimilate 40-45% of our food. This is about the maximum as the rest is fiber.

We should drink one ounce of water per pound of average body weight. Don't forget our body is 75-80% water so we need to replace that liquid every day. The purest water you can drink. But remember when you are drinking the vegetable juices this is the distilled water of the plant. They have water in them so that takes the place of your water. All disease is caused by toxemia which stems from the colon. We need to help the colon eliminate the body's waste products. We need to drink at least 3 qts. of vegetable juice a day. The inorganic minerals and wastes will be drawn out of the body thru the kidneys and the colon. To cleanse the colon we need to get the liver working.

Colonics will get the fecal matter out of the colon but it leaves the same weakened bowel area that was there before. Like an old inner tube that weakened bowel area balloons out. We need to get to the cause and clean up the bowel with herbs that heal and get the peristaltic motion going again. These foods or herbs feed and clean up the bowel so it will be healed and then it takes care of itself once it is well.

Dr. John Christopher has a lower bowel formula which heals the bowel and allows the muscles to go back in place after months of working with it. Depending on the person's bowel structure it may take 6-9 months to clean out the fecal matter from all the folds of the colon and to rebuild the bowel structure sufficiently to have the peristaltic muscles work on their own. You need to get the muscles to work properly so the prolapsed colon will go back into place. The lower bowel formula contains the following herbs which all have a work to do. Barberry works on the liver to get the bile flowing.[22] If the bile flows it works as a laxative. The barberry loosens hardened congealed bile so it will flow freely.

It may be in the form of little marbles or gallstones. We need to loosen this up. The liver needs this help so the colon will work properly. Then we use Cascara Sagrada. It is a specific food for the peristaltic muscle. It may have been dormant for years but this will reactivate it. Cayenne is a stimulant for the cell structure throughout the bowel. It will stop any bleeding if there are any problems there. Ginger acts as a leader to get all the other herbs into the abdominal area. It stops griping. Fennel helps to get rid of gas in the colon. It is an anti-colic herb, too. Lobelia is the thinking herb. Red Raspberry leaves bring back the iron the body needs. Turkey Rhubarb is a mild laxative. It can even be given to a baby. Goldenseal is the healing herb to rid the body of infection. This combination is a healing group of herbs. Start with 2 capsules three times a day. Use as many capsules as you need to get free flowing not formed bowel movements 3-5 times a day. One lady needed 40 capsules a

---

[22] The gall bladder stores the bile and secretes it as needed. If you have no gall bladder avoid all free fats and use proteins in moderation because your body can't handle them and it will make a lot of mucus. This includes beans, nuts, and seeds. Flaxseed oil is okay because it is an essential fatty acid the body uses. Don't heat it, though.

day to blast loose. You need to use Dr. Christopher's Fen LB formula. You may need to take this for 6 months to 1 year to heal the bowel. I have all of Dr. Christopher's herbs.

If you have a prolapsed colon you need extra help so it will go back into place. You need to use a slant board in the morning. Make a concentrated tea of oak bark, mullein, yellow dock, walnut leaves, comfrey root, lobelia, marshmallow root. You can order this at your health food store. It is called Dr. Christopher's Yellow Dock combination. Simmer down to one half its amount. Inject with a syringe into vagina one half-one cup of the cold tea or you can inject one pint into the rectum with a syringe or enema bag. You can hold it longer if cold because it causes the bowel to contract and it allows it to soak in. Leave this in as long as possible at least 20 minutes. Knead and massage the pelvic and abdominal area while on the slant board. Work it thru the whole ascending colon area then do a circular, clockwise massage. Work from the ascending colon up across the transverse colon down the descending colon into the sigmoid and out as you massage. Catnip tea is excellent to use by itself as it is a relaxing tea. You could alternate with these two teas. It is a nervine and it will cause the bowel to relax so you can break more fecal matter loose in the massage. Do not do any heavy massage to cause pain. As you find heavy fecal matter deposits in the colon work them loose with gentle massage. Inject no more than a pint into the rectum because you can't hold any more at one time. Remember the muscles are so weak in a prolapsed colon that they can't hold the bowel up. The bowel sags and more and more fecal matter collects in these folds where it hangs down. The fecal matter catches in the pockets. The colon balloons out. The herbal foods build up tissue and muscle. This helps a tipped uterus and problems in the reproductive organs because of a prolapsed transverse colon. A prolapsed colon can pinch the bladder & cause serious problems, such as when you laugh or sneeze you void some urine. This can be very embarrassing. So it is important to heal the colon and stimulate the muscles so the colon will go back in place. Use an injection of the combination herbs as above. Knead and massage while you hold the tea in the colon and the bowel will start to lift itself and go back into place again. It may not go back 100%, but it will help a great deal. Doing this will pay off if you have problems with the female reproductive organs, you can avoid surgery once everything goes back into place. The slant board routine and the FenLB capsules will help the male reproductive organs. They cleanse the prostate, too. There are many problems of the colon. A person can have a spastic colon, diverticula, strictures, prolapsed colon, etc.

Bleeding of the Colon can be a very frightening experience. When the first sign of blood is seen in the stool we tend to think the worst. It may be very serious but let's see what can be done to stop the bleeding. We use the herb mullein in a powdered form, but it needs to stick to the walls of the colon to stop the hemorrhaging. The best glue is made from cow's milk because it has 20 times more casein than the body can assimilate so it is left to be accepted in the form of glue on the walls of the colon. They use cow's milk to make Elmer's glue because it is so sticky. Any other time we would not want this extra coating on the colon walls but we need to get the mullein to stick there so it can stop the bleeding. Cow's milk is the only thing that will make the powdered mullein stay on the walls of the colon. You take one ounce of mullein and slow simmer it in one pint of whole cow's milk for 5 minutes. Strain it and drink the whole pint after each bowel movement. A certain man was put in the hospital by his family because he was losing great amounts of blood from the colon. He had various other health problems so they couldn't operate on him. They couldn't do anything to stop the bleeding so they were giving him continuous blood transfusions. The family and the gentleman were getting very discouraged. Someone suggested they take him to see Dr. John Christopher. They had him well padded when he was taken to see Dr. Christopher and he was taken into his office immediately. Dr. Christopher ask his secretary to go across the street and buy some cow's milk and make the milk and mullein mixture.

He went to the bathroom and then drank the pint of mullein and milk. The family was given the instructions on how to make it and that he was to drink one pint after each bowel movement. He followed this program throughout the day and by night the bleeding had stopped.

It is important that you continue this for one or two days more to assure complete stoppage of bleeding from the colon area. Drink the pint of milk and mullein mixture after each bowel movement. The third day drink it three times a day. Eat fruits, vegetables, whole grains, seeds, and nuts. After following this for one year you may want to clean the glue off the colon walls so the foods can be assimilated properly. Dr. Christopher has several herbal formulations for this. He has a FenLB or Cascara Sagrada which cleanse the colon. You need to do it faithfully for at least 6 months. Hemorrhoids are swellings of dilatation of veins surrounding the anus. They sometimes bleed and are almost always painful.

White oak bark, mullein, and bayberry are astringents or drawing herbs. You can make a strong tea by simmering to one half the volume you started with as, for example, if you had one quart you simmer it to one pint. Insert one pint of a cold infusion into the rectum with an enema bag or syringe. Lay on a slant board and hold it for 15-20 minutes so it can be assimilated. Drink three cups of the white oak bark tea a day. Use one half cup of the strong tea and dilute it with one half cup of distilled water. The white oak, bayberry, and mullein are very rich in organic calcium to feed the veins and arteries.

Many people have hemorrhoids that at times may bleed. You can make a suppository with the white oak bark, powdered and olive oil or vegetable glycerine. Work this into a pie dough consistency so it rolls easily in your fingers. Roll this into one and one half inch sizes. Keep in a plastic bag in the freezer until needed. Just before bed insert a peeled garlic bulb, dipped in olive oil, into the rectum as far up as it will go. Then insert the white oak suppository. These will come out with the first bowel movement in the morning. The garlic, bayberry, and the white oak are rich in organic calcium. This feeds the area the organic calcium to rebuild the veins and arteries. The white oak and bayberry are astringents so they pull the tissues back up into place. The garlic kills the infection. Taking a teaspoon of cayenne internally will stop the bleeding piles and feed and nourish the veins and arteries, too. Remember any sugar we eat in the form of sweets leaches the calcium out of the body and weakens the veins, arteries, and capillaries so they balloon out or rupture very easily. We can have weakened vein structure as in the form of piles, varicose veins, phlebitis, polyps, aneurisms, etc. They are all a shortage of organic calcium which we get from fruits, vegetables, whole grains, nuts, and seeds.

Dr. Christopher had a patient who had hemorrhoids that hung down five inches. He had to wear a truss to hold them in place. He began using the program as outlined in this paper. He detoxified the colon with LB formula. He took lots of cayenne and used LG formula for detoxifying the liver. His hemorrhoids went back into place and stayed there. Years later he had no hemorrhoids as long as he followed the mucusless diet. Remember it took a long time for the condition to develop so it won't go away over night. Follow the program faithfully.

THE LIVER

The liver is a large (3-4 pounds in an adult) glandular multipurpose organ located under the ribs on the right side beneath the diaphragm. It consists of two main lobes separated by a ligament.

Its weight can reach seven pounds but if so that would mean it (the liver) is very sick. It can also atrophy and become very small. Either one of these conditions means the liver needs cleansing.

The liver has many functions, including:

1. The manufacture and secretion of bile salts for emulsification and absorption of fats.
2. The conversion of sugar into glycogen, which it stores.
3. The manufacture of plasma proteins.
4. The formation of urea.
5. The storage of vitamins A, D, E, and K, iron and copper.
6. The activation of Vitamin D.
7. The supplier of enzymes which break down poisons or convert them into less harmful products.
8. The storage of poisons which cannot be broken down and excreted (Example: poisons from sprayed fruits and vegetables; drugs).

The liver receives a double supply of oxygenated and deoxygenated blood, containing newly absorbed nutrients. The nutrients are stored and used to make new materials. The poisons are stored or detoxified. Nutrients needed by other cells are secreted back into the blood. The liver draws the poisons from the pituitary gland, pineal gland, thyroid gland, reproductive organs, et cetera, just as a magnet attracts metal. The liver is, in effect, the cesspool of the body. The liver neutralizes these poisons which are converted into liver bile. The liver makes the bile which is then transferred to the gall bladder for concentration and elimination by the colon.

If you have a good lymph system, the poisons taken into the body go directly to the liver for neutralization. If the lymph system is kept clean and the bile is flowing properly, it means the liver is working well. As long as ten percent of the liver is still functioning, it can be reactivated with a detoxifying program and a rebuilding with herbs and vegetable juices. The liver (like the pancreas) is connected to the small intestine by a series of ducts. Often the liver breaks down and you get sick. Depending on where the weakness is in your body, you may have high blood pressure, cataracts, kidney disease, arteriosclerosis, cancer, et cetera. The enzyme system, immune system, insulin balance, hormone and mineral balance are all based in the liver. The liver is involved in all our chemical activities in the body. We have to help the liver if we are going to heal the body of chronic disease. A sick pancreas and a sick liver can't break down protein and this partially digested protein feeds cancer and causes all the other crippling and killer diseases.

You need a digest aid to digest the proteins and fats for you because the pancreas isn't working well. See information on Digest at end of booklet. Eliminate from your diet the meats, dairy products, processed foods, concentrated starches such as pastas, spaghetti, macaroni, et cetera, until you heal the liver. Fruits and vegetables, whole grains, seeds and nuts (unsalted, of course) until the crisis is past. Eat no fried foods, only baked or lightly steamed with a vegetable salad every day. Brown rice, artichokes and oatmeal are excellent foods to eat for nourishment, too. When the liver is so weak it can't handle fried foods, they clog the liver and weaken it still further. Once your liver is restored, hopefully you will continue to follow a healthy diet.

The diseased cells die when you put potassium into the body, which are the live vital enzymes rich in oxidative materials. You need to give the liver the help it needs to get rid of these dead cells so they can be eliminated from the body. Detoxify the liver as the tumor tissue is broken down. The cells die and must be expelled. If you don't do this, the liver can go into a coma because you get self-intoxicated. You must detoxify the liver. Barberry and cayenne or Dr. Christopher's Red Clover Combination formula are good for the liver.

You may get a healing reaction when you start on a natural healing program. The body will do its best to fight the disease and in the process, you may become nauseous, get a fever, et cetera. This a signal to detoxify with Dr. Christopher's FenLB or Lower Bowel herbal formula. You can slow down this healing and cleansing process by eating cooked food. Do under the care of a natural healing doctor.

Liver Weaknesses

The liver can become enlarged because of too many poisons and toxins. It may become jaundiced, and the skin and eyes take on a yellow color. Infectious hepatitis of liver is caused by a virus. It is spread by contamination. It can produce chronic liver inflammation. One form of hepatitis can be spread by blood transfusion. These could become more severe, so it is necessary to detoxify the liver. Any enlargement of the liver is an infection which means too many toxins and poisons Meat protein damages the liver and the kidneys, too. It depends on how good your liver and kidneys are before you suffer disease because of poisons produced from animal proteins.

MEDICAL DIAGNOSIS OF LIVER PROBLEMS

Please note the following medical profession approach for diagnosing the liver:

"Clinical Application: Liver tissue for diagnostic purposes may be obtained by performing a liver biopsy. In the procedure, the needle is inserted through the 7th, 8th or 9th intercostal space while the person is holding his or her breath in full expiration. This lessens the possibility of damage to the lung and contamination of the pleural cavity."[23]

The above "Clinical Application" procedure and the fact that biopsies themselves are known to spread cancer are the reasons I do not recommend ever having any kind of biopsy!!

Cleansing the Liver

The liver is the principal organ in the body which can remain deteriorated for many years before its great functional reserves are consumed. Conversely, the liver has a great capacity to heal, to regenerate itself. However, once those functional reserves are consumed, self-healing may not be possible, and the liver has to be cleansed. One tenth of the liver may be functioning and you can reactivate the rest if you are willing to follow a health program.

There are differing methods for cleansing the liver: Juices, herbs, castor oil packs, and muscular movement and deep breathing to get the lymphatic system to work properly.

---

[23]   *Principles of Anatomy and Physiology*, G. Lortora and N. Anagnostakos, p 606.

Liver Herbs

The herbs used for liver cleansing include milk thistle, dandelion, barberry (also called maiden barber) and wild yam, along with blue flag, cayenne, chickweed, comfrey, juniper, Oregon grape, chaparral and purple loosestrife.[24]

Barberry is an old Indian remedy for the digestive system and the liver (as well as the gall bladder). Dr. Ratner, a famous herbalist, believed that barberry was one of the best herbs for stimulating the liver, especially in cases of jaundice, where it can soften and break up congealed bile and cause it to flow through the gall bladder into the digestive tract.

Dr. Christopher agreed, for barberry was the main herb which he used as part of a powerful liver-GB formula to cleanse and purify the liver.[25] Barberry is probably unequaled as a corrector of liver secretions (and it causes the bile to flow more freely) while it expels and removes morbid waste material from the stomach and bowels.[26]

Barberry also regulates the digestive system, lessens the size of the spleen and removes obstructions in the intestinal tract.

One reason barberry is so effective in purifying the liver is that it contains a high content of a substance called berberine. Dr. Christopher did a chemical analysis of barberry and found that the amount of berberine was 5.37 percent. However, berberine should not be extracted from barberry and taken in solution. While berberine cleans out the bile and is thus an invaluable herb in maintaining health throughout the body, the rest of the minerals in barberry act as a catalyst to make the berberine work so much better. Both the barberry berries and the root bark of the herb are used but the root bark possesses the more powerful medicinal properties.

Liver treatments will depend upon the state of the liver to be treated, as well as the individual's overall condition. If the person is relatively strong but suffers from severe liver problems, then he or she should receive castor oil packs. If the person with liver problems is in a very weakened condition, he

---

[24] Dr. Christopher's Liveron capsules will cleanse the liver.

[25] The formula consists of barberry, wild yam, cramp bark, fennel seed, ginger, catnip and peppermint. It is taken by capsule twice daily.

[26] Barberry root bark, in large concentrated doses, can purge, so mild doses should be taken until natural elimination results. Barberry acts as a laxative, aiding assimilation by eliminating toxic build-up in the intestine. It will help to remove intestinal obstructions. Diarrhea will also respond to the berries of barberry.

or she should not go on an intensive program without the supervision of a doctor. Do the castor oil packs once a day till you see how they do.

For severe liver conditions, take the milder herbs to first calm down the system so it can handle the cleansing. Start by cleansing the colon with Dr. Christopher's FenLB or Lower Bowel formula. Take enough capsules to move the colon three times a day (see the Colon section). Some people have to start with 2 capsules at night and increase as needed. Drink two quart of carrot juice a day.

Lymphatic System

The lymphatic system needs to be working well so the liver can detoxify and get rid of the poisons. Oregon grape herb and cayenne are good for the lymphatic system. The lymphatic system needs to carry away the poisons released from the liver.

Milk Thistle and Dandelion

Milk thistle and dandelion are important herbs for a diseased liver yet mild enough to serve as the first step in the cleansing process. This is of particular concern if the person's condition is delicate. Dandelion root lowers high blood sugar.

Begin slowly to cleanse the liver with a milk thistle and dandelion tea. Drink at least four cups a day to detoxify the liver.

Barberry and Wild Yam Teas

For jaundice, hepatitis or other liver problems, use three parts of barberry and one part wild yam (or two parts of sweet fennel). Take one half cup every hour of the barberry and wild yam during the day (take one quart or more of carrot juice, also, during the day), as often as the person can tolerate it during the day. This will start the liver working and may be used along with the castor oil packs.

To make the tea heat the water to boiling and take one level teaspoon of barberry and wild yam mixture per cup. Let steep for thirty minutes and drink. Incidently, don't worry if your skin turns yellow as this is okay, it is the bile being freed rapidly. Sixty percent of our poisons are eliminated through the skin so when the bile can't get out fast enough through the kidneys and colon, the bile will take the next best route. We save ourselves a lot of grief by detoxifying the liver with the liver herbs regularly before it gets into a crisis situation.

CASTOR OIL PACKS

Treat the liver externally twice daily with castor oil packs. Start by massaging olive oil into the liver area for five minutes each day.

This goes in to heal and rebuild new tissue. Before you do the castor oil pack each day rub in olive oil. Then you are ready for the castor oil pack. Dip a white cloth in castor oil, removing excess oil, and cover the liver area. Cover with plastic. Put an electric heating pad on it and relax for 30 minutes to one hour. You may use a hot water bottle if you wish, if you don't have a heating pad. If you have a severe condition it is good to put a cold pack on the liver using cold water from the tap. Place this cold pack on the liver for 5 minutes and then go back to the castor oil pack for 30 minutes. Alternate back & forth with the hot and cold packs. The castor oil goes into the liver area and lymph glands, draws out poisons and flushes the poisons as tumors, cysts, or polyps out of the body. All drugs, prescription or non-prescription, are liver toxic. Any drugs you have taken in your life can be stored for years, and the liver becomes overloaded and overworked. Be good to your liver—flush it.

Dr. John Christopher had a patient who had just come home from the hospital with only a few days to live. The lady had hepatitis of the liver. Her skin was yellow and so were the whites of her eyes. She was in very heavy pain. Dr. Christopher started her on barberry and wild yam tea. She drank one half cup every hour or so throughout the day. She did the castor oil packs on the liver. They kept her on juices with most of it being carrot juice. In a few days she was feeling much better. Dr. Christopher saw her six years later and she was full of pep and energy. Her liver was functioning well.

If you have a liver with many cancerous tumors I would do the castor oil pack about every two hours and follow the rest of the program for the liver plus the rest of the system. If the liver is swollen several times its size it is saying help me detoxify. The liver will restore itself with the proper help as per this book. Don't use the cloth but once. Have an old white sheet you can tear into the right size.

THE SKIN

The skin is the body's largest eliminative organ which eliminates sixty percent of all our poisons. Nutrients as in liquid herbs placed on the skin, or the use of fomentations, can be absorbed through the skin. If a person can't swallow you can rub the liquid herbs on the throat area, for example. We have an acid mantle flora on our skin which keeps the invaders out. Use of harsh soaps can clog the millions of pores so the poisons are reabsorbed back into the body to do damage elsewhere in the body. The skin is our second set of kidneys so be good to your skin.

Miracle 2 all natural soap is a biodegradable, nontoxic soap. Its use after dry-skin brushing (use a natural bristle brush) just before your bath gets the lymph flowing, increases the circulation, cleanses the skin of the dead cells and restores the skin's ability to eliminate. The Miracle 2 soap is a great shampoo as well as a soap for cleansing the body. It may be used to replace all of your chemical cleaning products.

CAYENNE PEPPER

Cayenne (or capsicum) is a medicinal and nutritional herb. It is the purest and most certain stimulant. This herb is a great food for the circulatory system in that it feeds the necessary elements into the cell structure of the arteries, veins, and capillaries so that these regain the elasticity of youth again, and the blood pressure adjusts itself to normal. Cayenne is a fruit belonging to the Solanaceae family of 5 species and 300 varieties of plants that produce fleshy vegetable pods called capsicums. It contains capsaicin which gives it its stimulating action. African Cayenne is the most potent along with the Indian Cayenne. Cayenne's potency is measured in heat units. African Cayenne has 90,000 or more heat units. Cayenne is rich in Vitamins A, B, C, B1, B2, and B12, zinc and niacin. It contains organic calcium, potassium, iron, magnesium, phosphorus, selenium, other nutrients. It rebuilds the tissue in the stomach and heals stomach and intestinal ulcers, in equalizing the blood circulation. Cayenne produces natural warmth: and in stimulating the peristaltic motion of the intestines, it aids in assimilation and elimination. Cayenne is first aid for strokes and heart attacks and relieves the angina pains because it increases the circulation of the blood to the heart muscle.

When the venous structure becomes loaded with sticky mucus, the blood has a harder time circulating; therefore higher pressure forces the liquid through. Cayenne regulates the flow of blood from the head to the feet so that it is equalized; it influences the heart immediately, then gradually extends its effects to the arteries, capillaries, and nerves. (The frequency of the pulse is not increased, but is given more power.) If there is an external or internal wound one teaspoon of Cayenne in one cup of warm water will stop the bleeding by the time you count to ten. It equalizes the blood pressure from the top of the head to the feet so this keeps the pressure from the hemorrhage area so it will clot naturally.

Cayenne needs to be used generously when there is a circulation problem. Take capsules if you can't take the powder. The quickest way to get it into the system is stir-1 tsp. Cayenne into some thick juice and drink it. Always take Cayenne on a full stomach except in an emergency situation as it may cause some burning as it is so stimulating and it may make you feel faint when it begins its work that is because it is such a stimulant to the system. You may want to drink some peppermint tea along with it. They both work well together. Always start slow so you may want to try ½ teaspoon of cayenne to some thick juice.

Cayenne stimulates the liver and gall bladder to promote the flow of bile. Cayenne is the best food for the circulation. A stroke patient has a circulation problem. Cayenne reduces the mucus in all body systems and the result is good circulation. Cayenne is a circulatory stimulant. If you have a burning sensation when you take it, don't give up. It means you need it badly. It is trying to correct something in your body. Dr. Christopher says to eat a piece of bread and drink some water to move it along and the burning will stop.

Here is a true story about the phenomenal powers of Cayenne to increase circulation. It is taken from a rare book entitled, "The Healing Miracles of Cayenne Pepper." In 1870 there was a lumberjack named James McCann, a young man who started to go back to the states by way of California. He reached Parowan with both feet frozen above his ankles. He was left with me (Dr. Meeks) to have both feet amputated as it was thought there was no possible chance to save his life without amputation. An impulse seemed to strike my mind as though by inspiration that I would give him Cayenne Pepper inwardly and see what effect that would have on the frozen feet. "I commenced by giving him rather small doses at first, one teaspoon at a time. It increased the warmth and power of the action of the blood to such a degree that it gave him such pain and misery in his legs that he could not bear it. He laid down on his back and elevated his feet up against the wall for three or four days so he could sit up in a chair.

The new flesh would form as fast as the dead flesh would get out of the way. In fact, the new flesh would seem to crowd the dead flesh.

That was all the medical treatment he had and to my astonishment and that of everyone else who knew of the circumstances, the 16th day after I gave him the first dose of Cayenne, he walked nine miles from Parowan to Red Creek and back. Both his feet were saved! He lost but five toenails.

Cayenne purifies the blood. I am convinced that there is nothing like Cayenne and you will find it applicable in all cases of sickness."[27]

One of the most common herbal uses of Cayenne is as a gastric stimulant and digestive aid. It rebuilds the stomach tissue and stimulates peristalsis. Thus it is very helpful in assimilation and elimination. The natives in the West Indies don't fear the deadly yellow fever—as long as they have a good supply of Cayenne! Cayenne heals ulcers.

Cayenne (powdered) taken in some liquid and given to a heart attack victim brings them out of the heart attack within about 2 minutes. The Cayenne expands the cell walls, goes directly to the heart and stimulates it to beat properly. Dr, Christopher's advice for someone who has suffered a heart attack, if they are conscious do the following. Prepare one teaspoon of Cayenne in a cup of warm water.

Prop up the person and have them drink quite quickly the cayenne tea. The heart attack will stop in about two minutes.[28] Important: Make sure the person is able to swallow it.

Here is another testimony to Cayenne's powers. Doctors wanted to remove part of a man's stomach. He had a severe case of stomach ulcers. One night he came home from work sick enough to die. He was in great pain. He took a heaping tablespoon of Cayenne in a glass of warm water and gulped it down. Then he made a discovery which made him very happy. He found his wife was correct about herbs.

Cayenne soon stopped his stomach pains for the first time in months. He fell asleep and he slept all night. He awoke with no pain. This was the first time he had no pain in months. He kept taking three teaspoons each day, and soon his stomach ulcers were gone. Cayenne regulates blood pressure & cleans the blood.

Dr. Christopher said, "When I was 35, the doctors said I would be dead by age 43." Dr. Christopher had advanced hardening of the arteries. His veins would stick out of his hands like pencils. He had crippling arthritis, stomach ulcers and was the victim of two horrible automobile accidents. He started taking Cayenne Pepper in warm water three times a day and he did this for ten years. He went for a physical when he was 45. When the doctor took his blood pressure it was perfectly normal. One medical doctor told him, "I see your age is 45, but you have the venous structure of a teenage boy. I've

[27]   Dr. John R. Christopher's newsletter, *Health Discoveries*, Issue Number 17.

[28]   Dr. John R. Christopher - School of Natural Healing.

never seen anything like it!" "The healing power of nature is in the blood. To accelerate the blood is to accelerate the healing power of nature."[29]

Do not use Cayenne (red pepper) from the grocery store. This is not the herb and it is an irritant to the system. It is an inorganic spice which has been irradiated. Only purchase the Cayenne from your health provider.

With cayenne you may notice a more positive attitude, less procrastination, longer periods between rest, sounder sleep, bowel regularity, improved appetite, freedom from headache, muscle cramps, an enhanced sense of health & well being. Cayenne has been known to relieve all body systems with proper nutrition & detoxification. It has relieved paralyzed conditions of strokes, even if the person has been in a wheelchair.

Dr. Richard Schultz tells about seeing a patient have a stroke in his waiting room. He says he saw his blood vessels enlarge and then explode in front of him. Then the person fell to the floor. Dr. Schultz gave him 10 dropperfuls of cayenne tincture and he came out of the stroke right away. He left the office on his own. If you don't have the tincture give them a tablespoon of cayenne powder in warm water especially if they are having a heart attack, too. This goes right to the heart and stimulates the heart to beat properly. Dr. Schultz recommends 1 tablespoon of cayenne powder three times a day for a few days after the stroke. Then stay on a teaspoon of cayenne powder three-four times a day. Dr. Christopher got results with a teaspoon of cayenne in a cup of warm water for a heart attack victim.

Cayenne is for heart and blood circulation problems, angina pains, palpitations, cardiac arrhythmia and it is great for congestive heart failure along with Dr. John Christopher's Hawthorn berry syrup. It is specific for any circulatory problem, such as high or low blood pressure, triglycerides and fats, varicose veins, etc. You need to stay on a mucusless diet, too.

You can give babies cayenne tincture in their bottle and save their life if they have any breathing problems. A newborn that had asthma was saved by a few drops of cayenne tincture every day in a bottle of liquid. Don't ever be without a good cayenne powder it may save a loved one's life. Cayenne stimulates the cerebral circulation so it helps if someone is faint or going to pass out. Cayenne stops any unnatural bleeding.

---

[29] For additional reading on Cayenne, see *Back to Eden* by Jethro Kloss, pages 215-230.

CHELATION THERAPY

Inorganic calcium builds up on the arteries and blood vessels so the blood can't get through as it should. This causes the heart to pump harder and the blood becomes thicker, et cetera. We then have high blood pressure, high cholesterol, arteriosclerosis, a stroke, heart disease, diabetes, et cetera. There are too many fats circulating in the blood and being deposited on the arteries and blood vessels. You need the Omega 3, essential fatty acids, found in flaxseed oil to hold the other oils in suspension so they can be gotten out of the body properly so they aren't deposited on arteries and blood vessels. Essential fatty acids are present in walnuts, toasted wheat germ, olives and flaxseed.[30]

A stroke is the result of blood pressure in the brain caused by impurities in the blood vessels as inorganic calcium caused by eating excessive amounts of starches and rich foods over a period of years. This causes impaction in the lower intestines with the consequent absorption of toxins.[31]

Organic calcium's effect on cholesterol levels is that it acts as a normalizer. Adequate organic calcium found in vegetables, fruits, grain, seeds and nuts protects us from strokes, heart disease, et cetera.

Chelation Therapy is very important to remove these deposits. If you find a natural healing doctor, he may do I.V. chelation. Be good to yourself start a program. Chelation therapy solves many different problems where there is inorganic calcium on the blood vessels and arteries or inorganic aluminum on the brain. Talk to your natural healing doctor. If you can't find one in your area I have a list of them by states. I would advise you to read Bypassing the Bypass by Elmer Cranston along with other books on chelation therapy you

---

[30] Don't heat the flaxseed oil as this makes it harmful.

[31] N.W. Walker, *Fresh Vegetable and Fruit Juices*, p. 112.

may find at your local health food store or library. I have a list of natural healing doctors by states if you are interested in finding one please contact me.

You may have a blockage of blood vessels by plaque which reduces the flow of blood, thus starving the vital organs of oxygen and other minerals and nutrients for survival. The cell walls may become leaky and this allows excessive calcium, sodium, and other elements to enter. Inorganic Calcium deposits may form and harden. These cause coronaries and other arteries to go into spasm and reduce the blood flow to vital organs. Plaques are composed of fibrous tissue, cholesterol and calcium. Atherosclerosis is caused by these accumulations of plaque. They block the flow of blood. Atherosclerosis leads to heart attack, stroke, senility and could lead to amputation of limbs unless you follow God's methods of healing using diet and herbs.

Chelation therapy is a safe, effective and relatively inexpensive way to restore blood flow without surgery. Chelation therapy is the intravenous infusion of product called EDTA. EDTA removes undesirable metals from the body which have been deposited on the arteries and blood vessels or been deposited in the brain, such as inorganic aluminum which is the cause of Alzheimer disease. EDTA improves calcium and cholesterol metabolism by eliminating metallic catalysts which cause damage to cell membranes by producing "free radicals." Free radical pathology is an important contributing cause of atherosclerosis, cancer, diabetes, and other diseases of aging. EDTA helps to prevent the production of harmful free radicals.

Chelation therapy corrects the major underlying cause of arterial blockage. EDTA removes metallic irritants allowing the leaky and damaged cell walls to heal. It shrinks and removes the plaque so more blood can flow thru. It makes the arterial walls softer and more pliable so the walls can expand easier. The blood flow is increased throughout your body so you have increased circulation.

When you take Chelation Therapy you also need to follow a good nutritional program of only fruits, vegetables, whole grains, seeds, and nuts. Eliminate processed foods, sweets, meats and dairy products for the best results. A program of regular exercise, vitamin and mineral supplementation and avoidance of alcohol and tobacco is important. You can get your minerals and vitamins by doing fresh raw vegetable juice every day. Green Star is very versatile. You can even make your own ice cream with frozen fruit. Take Chatfield's powdered carob and mix it with nut milk for a nice "chocolate" syrup made of carob & add some honey. It is delicious. I am a distributor for Green Star. You can make your own whole wheat noodles, juice wheatgrass & other leafy vegetables, make fruit juice. It has a 5 year warranty on the motor.

It triturates so you have the hydrogen peroxide molecule in tact. You can't have normal cell division without the hydrogen peroxide molecule. It runs at only 110 RPM. Green Star triturates the veggies into a pulp by splitting open the cells of the fibers thus liberating the live enzymes which are readily & quickly assimilated by the body. They are rich in potassium & they are live enzymes so they quickly regenerate.

Chelation is a natural process in your body. When your body needs extra iron somewhere, the iron molecules are bonded (chelated) with the natural chelating material hemoglobin in the blood. Once it is chelated with the hemoglobin, the iron is then carried throughout the body and used where it is needed.

Alfred Werner a French-Swiss chemist originated the idea of intravenous chelation in 1893. He discovered that natural chelators could be introduced to remove poisons and toxins. Compared to bypass surgery (doesn't solve heart problems) but accounts for thousands of deaths every year, more than one million people have reaped the healing benefits of IV Chelation since 1954 with not one single death.

Chelation Therapy requires numerous doctor visits and takes several hours each time. It is much cheaper than bypass surgery and requires hardly any pain. All you have is the prick of the needle as the IV is inserted in the arm. You can then relax and listen to relaxing music or visit with the other patients.

The word chelation is taken from the Greek word chele which means "claw." This represents the way a natural chelation formula, made up of specific antioxidants, vitamins, minerals, and herbs, moves through your blood and "grabs" certain harmful substances and escorts them out of your body.

Remember the body can only use organic products. It will accept inorganic products such as the inorganic calcium in milk and dairy products but it will deposit them on the arteries and blood vessels causing high blood pressure, high cholesterol, plaque on the arteries, heart disease, strokes, etc. We need to get our calcium naturally from carrot juice, vegetables eaten raw in a salad, seeds, and nuts so the body can assimilate it.

Chelation restores the structural integrity of your arteries and protects against heart problems. It removes the deadly deposits that cause problems, renews the cells that line your arteries, and restores their flexibility. You will find renewed energy and stamina. Your arteries and blood are swept clean and you won't run out of breath as often. Your arteries become more flexible and elastic. Your blood flows more freely without taxing the heart. Your blood pressure is restored to normal. Dangerous inorganic calcium deposits are removed, thus lowering your risk of a heart attack. You can live a longer, healthier life. There are so many benefits we couldn't begin to name them all. Some other benefits are ward off senility, improve vision, fight osteoporosis, avoid gallstones, improve kidney function, maintain healthy blood sugar levels, relieve breathing problems, etc.

Remember you don't have to become another victim. You don't have to be another statistic. You don't have to worry about the side effects of drugs. You don't have to submit to painful and deadly bypass surgery. God has a better way.

FLAXSEED OIL

Flaxseed Oil is a clear, moderately-viscous oil derived from pressed flax seeds. It contains high quality, easily digestible and complete protein, all of the amino acids essential to human health and in good balance. The essential amino acids cannot be made by the human body and must therefore be provided through the diet. If all the essential amino acids are supplied, our bodies can manufacture from them the other dozen or so amino acids required to make all of our proteins. If any one or more essential amino acids is missing from the diet, protein deficiency disease develops.[32]

A few of the functions of essential fatty acids follow:

1. They are essential components, along with proteins, in the structure of every cell wall & internal cell components.
2. They are required for energy production & oxidation in the body.
3. They are essential for sperm formation for conception.
4. They are essential in the foetus for brain & nerve formation & in human mother's milk for continued brain & nerve growth. Cow's milk as in baby formulas, is almost devoid of essential fatty acids. These deficiencies are strongly implicated in learning disabled children.
5. Essential fatty acids increase the ease of dissolving body fat into body fluids. Therefore, they can remove arteriosclerosis & permit good weight control.
6. Their deficiencies appear to be important factors in most human illness.[33]

---

[32] *Fats and Oils, The Complete Guide to Fats and Oils in Health and Nutrition*, P. 264, by Udo Erasmus.

[33] *Fats and Oils, ibid.*

We are what we eat—plus air & water. You can't make healthy blood if you don't eat live food.

There are 45 essential nutrients which we need. They are broken down into 15 vitamins, 20 minerals, 8 essential amino acids (building blocks for proteins) & 2 essential fatty acids (linoleic & linolenic acid). We don't hear much about the essential fatty acids. We need all of them every day. Twenty nine of these are involved in fat metabolism. Seventy eight percent of the Americans die because of degenerative disease such as cardiovascular disease, cancer, multiple sclerosis, diabetes, or cystic fibrosis. All of them are fat metabolism problems. The body isn't breaking down the fats they are ingesting. The fat is being deposited on the arteries & blood vessels because they are getting too much of the saturated fat & not enough, if any, of the essential fatty acids.

There are many other degenerative diseases with a major fat metabolism problem; arthritis, PMS, osteoporosis, which is, also, a calcium problem. Don't take calcium supplements they won't solve it. You need raw vegetable juices, sesame seeds-ground, etc. Behavioral problems (schizophrenia, depression) respond to good nutrition & detoxifying the body. Degeneration of inner organs (liver, kidney, & brain) respond well to good nutrition. Cardiovascular disease is killing one in two.

You need the essential fatty acids everyday in order to be healthy. Your body doesn't manufacture them. You must obtain them from your food. The Omega 3 group is the linolenic acid. The richest source is flaxseed oil. Walnuts, toasted wheat germ, & soybeans have Omega 3. The Omega 6 is the linoleic acid. Polyunsaturated nuts & seeds contain Omega 6. If you don't eat some of these every day, your body begins to deteriorate. When your supply is totally used up you die.

What are the functions of the essential fatty acids? "First, essential fatty acids are required for the transport & metabolism of both cholesterol & triglycerides. They are able to lower high cholesterol levels by up to 25 percent & high triglyceride levels up to 65 percent.

"Second, essential fatty acids, & especially the Omega 3s, are required for normal development of the brain. In the adult, they are required for brain function. In the human foetus, brain development begins six weeks after conception, and is completed about one year after birth. In animal studies it has been shown that when the mother's diet is deficient in Omega 3 fatty acids, her adult offspring show permanent learning disabilities. We haven't done controlled experiments on human populations, but we know that Omega 3 fatty acids are required for human brain development, & if you think about the increasing incidence of learning disabilities of our school children, you might guess that we have a similar situation of Omega 3 deficiencies.

"In the adult, Omega 3s are required in visual function (retina), brain & nerve function (synapses), adrenal function (stress), & testis function (sperm formation). Clinical studies indicate that Omega 3s bring a sense of calmness. They interfere with the production of chemicals which the body makes in response to stress. They improve the behavior of schizophrenics & juvenile delinquents.

"Third, essential fatty acids & their derivatives are components required in the structure of the membranes that surround each cell in our body & each organelle (the little factories that carry on various specific cellular activities) within each cell. When we lack essential fatty acids, we end up with leaky membranes. Substances which ought not to pass in and out of cells, with several effects on the organism. The electrical potential of the cells is altered; vitality is lowered; gastrointestinal problems arise, skin afflictions occur and allergic reactions take place because foreign substances get into our body. Then, our immune system has to deal with it.

"Fourth, essential fatty acids stimulate metabolism, increase metabolic rate, increase oxygen uptake, & increase energy production. These effects can be measured on the cellular level. Oxidation & energy production are the most important moment to moment functions of every cell. They work through oxidation, molecules of food are broken down into carbon dioxide & water. Oxygen is a necessary part of that process. Energy is released during oxidation, & this energy is the energy our cells require to do their work on the molecular level. This energy is also our vitality, the energy we use to think, to act, & to accomplish."[34]

Essential fatty acids are oxygenated so they put oxygen in the body. This gives you more energy, almost immediately, especially if you are very low on the essential fatty acids. They slow down cancer cell growth & candida yeast growth. Disease can't live where there is oxygen. Deep breathe as often as you can to put oxygen in your system.

The body makes prostaglandins from the essential fatty acids. They make the blood platelets less sticky so they don't clump together. They regulate arterial muscle tone so the blood pressure goes down. It helps the arteries relax. They regulate inflammatory response. Prostaglandins help get rid of fluids

---

[34] *Fats and Oils, The Complete Guide to Fats and Oils in Health and Nutrition*, by Udo Erasmus.

in the body so you don't have water retention. They stimulate the immune system. Stress increases the bad PG2s which make sticky platelets, high blood pressure, edema, inflammation, & lowered immunity. Trust in God. Immune function needs the essential fatty acids to kill infectious organisms.

We need to avoid the hard fats in margarine, shortening oils, lard, dairy products, and palm kernel oil. These are dumped in the arteries and in the cells the form of fatty tumors. Stay away from fried foods. These increase the cancer we've seen in the past 80 years.

Research in 1888 has shown that starving dogs continued to deteriorate when fed animal protein and saturated fats. These dogs recovered rapidly, however, when they were fed both sulfur-rich vegetable proteins & good fresh flaxseed oil.

Dr. Johanna Budwig, who began her work with cancer about 1953, found the blood of cancer guests was deficient in the essential fatty acids. She found a yellow-green protein substance in the blood instead of the healthy red blood hemoglobin. This explained the anemia of cancer-an oxygen deficiency disease. The abnormal division of cancer cells can perhaps partly be explained as a deficiency of linoleic acid & sulfur rich proteins necessary for cell membrane production. Dr. Budwig found that with sulphur rich protein, fresh flaxseed oil and dietary improvements, within three months the yellow-green substance was replaced with red, vitality returned, proper lipoproteins & phosphatides appeared; anemia was alleviated; tumors receded & disappeared; & the person recuperated. Symptoms of cancer, diabetes, & liver disease disappeared.

There are many diseases of fatty degeneration. These degenerative diseases are caused by a lack of Vitamin C, B6, niacin, zinc and other minerals. For good health we need to eat fruits, vegetables, whole grains, seeds, & nuts. This supplies the body with the high potassium we need for each cell to function properly. We need potassium in the cells. The sodium is to stay in the blood serum. When we have disease the potassium leaks out of the cells & the sodium rushes in to fill the void. We then need to re-establish the balance with lots of potassium foods & fresh vegetable juices.[35]

Decrease your intake of non essential fats, cholesterol, & sugar (this forms hard fats & cholesterol on arteries) so you can prevent enzyme blocking. Your health is your responsibility not the doctor's. He only treats symptoms. Follow God's plan & He will bless.

---

[35] For more information, see *Fresh Vegetable and Fruit Juices* by NW Walker.

For optimum health you want the best. Barlean's Flaxseed Oil is pressed the day it is shipped. I have Barlean's at my Herb Shop. The Flaxseed Oil is organic and pesticide free. This is the purest & best. The Lignan rich flaxseed oil is the best source of nutrients. It contains about 55-65 percent alpha linolenic acid. Barlean's is interested in always manufacturing high quality oils with your health as their goal. Glass allows light to destroy the oil. Only buy it in the black containers. They stamp a date on it so you know it is fresh. Barlean's guarantees quality & freshness with their name. Put it on your salads or other fresh vegetables. The only symptom from getting too much flaxseed oil is extra energy. Most of us could use more of that.

Dr Budwig has worked with 1000 documented successful cancer cases in Germany. She uses whole grains, fresh vegetables & juices, fresh fruit, herbs & flaxseed oil with sulfur-rich protein. She uses no supplements with her guests. She has her cancer guests take about seven tablespoons of fresh flaxseed oil each day.

In summary, flaxseed oil helps.

1 Heart disease: Omega 3s lower blood cholesterol and triglyceride levels. This helps prevent a clot blocking an artery in the brain, heart attacks and pulmonary embolism.

2. Arthritis: This is a fat metabolism problem plus a build-up of uric acid. The body doesn't get enough essential fatty acids.

3. Cancer: The essential fatty acids in flaxseed oil dissolve tumors. Charlotte Gerson still uses flaxseed oil in a cancer treatment begun by her father, Dr. Max Gerson, in the 1950s. at her clinic in Mexico, with good results. Dr. Budwig considers the flaxseed oil, with a sulfur based protein, to be the most important ingredient in her cancer treatment.

4. Diabetes: This is a deficiency of Omega 3 and Omega 6 fatty acids. It is a fat metabolism problem so plaque builds up on arteries and blood vessels.

5. Asthma: This is relieved within a few days of taking the oil.

6. PMS: Many times, it relieves the problem in one month.

7. Allergies: Good nutrition with flaxseed oil as part of the program helps relieve allergy symptoms.

8. Inflammatory Tissue Disease: This includes the 'itis's as in tendinitis, bursitis, meningitis, et cetera.

9. Water Retention; This helps the kidneys take sodium and water out of the body. This helps edema, swollen ankles, et cetera.

10. It alleviates skin problems and gives you more energy.
11. Flaxseed oil helps multiple sclerosis. It puts the myelin sheath on the nerve cells. In cystic fibrosis, it loosens viscous mucous secretions and relieves breathing. Some behavioral problems as depression, schizophrenia and other pathologically deviant behaviors are relieved.

REGENERATION TEA (BFC)

Dr. Christopher has a combination called Regeneration Tea (BFC). It is very rich in calcium. It literally regenerates the body (bone, flesh, and cartilage).

Pour one gallon of best water into a stainless steel pot. Boil the water. Remove from heat. Add one half cup of the loose cut BFC Tea. If you want stronger tea, add more. Turn off the burner. Let it steep for one hour. Strain and drink at least six cups a day. Sweeten with honey. This tea rebuilds nerve, muscle, and bone tissues as well as any organ tissue in the body. BFC Tea purifies, builds up and regenerates the body. It is a miracle tea! For frozen shoulder or other locked joints or fluid on the elbow or knee place a hot fomentation[36] over the area with the BFC tea or Burdock root. Cover with plastic and leave on for 30 minutes at a time. Drink some of the tea, also. Take one fourth cup of the strong tea to three fourths of best water. Drink as much as you can. Do the hot fomentations until you get relief. See footnote for more information on fomentations. You may do 30 minutes of a hot fomentation and 5 minutes of cold for excellent results.

BFC tea is excellent for all types of degeneration of the body. It rebuilds marrow, bone, flesh, and cartilage. The tea contains the herbs oak bark, comfrey root, mullein, walnut leaves, marshmallow root, wormwood, lobelia, scullcap, and gravel root. Dr. Christopher's BFC salve heals cuts, wounds,

---

[36] Fomentations are applications of hot, moist cloths to the body to ease pain, increase circulation, carry away infection, etc. Fomentations are made by boiling one gallon of distilled water. Turn off the heat and add 3/4 cup of BFC Tea. Let the Tea soak for 4-6 hours. Turn on low heat and simmer to 1/4 the Tea's original volume, or one quart. Strain the liquid. This makes a strong tea for applying to the skin.

muscle strains, tendinitis, etc. Rub on three times a day. Apply the BFC Salve to a Plantar's wart, which has a center core, for at least two weeks.

The hardened outer shell and most of the center should come out leaving the inner core to come off. Then, apply Dr. Christopher's Black Salve and the core of the wart should come out.[37]

For skin cancer,[38] rub in Dr. Christopher's Deep Heating Cayenne Salve first. This increases circulation. Then apply the Black Salve.[39] One man had horrible skin cancer covering over 45 percent of his face. Two months after using the Cayenne Salve and Black Salve, it disappeared. The BFC Salve in combination with the Cayenne Salve will take the pain and inflammation out of arthritis and start to restore the body if you, also drink the BFC to wash the uric acid out of the body. See my literature for more information.

You may want to use powdered comfrey mixed with olive oil and made into a paste for skin ulcers, bunions, etc. Keep applying as it is absorbed each day so it stays moist on the area. It is high in potassium, calcium, magnesium, and protein. It is a cell proliferant. Powdered slippery elm is excellent for ulcers, bedsores, etc. made the same way. Use powdered comfrey, wheat germ oil, & honey in equal portions for 2nd & 3rd degree burns. Keep applying it & tape lightly. Never let it dry out.

---

[37] My daughter's wart on the bottom of her foot did just that and there was never a trace of it, again. It went away completely.

[38] The subject of cancer is covered extensively in the author's booklet on *Cancer and You.*

[39] Dr. Christopher said it has an almost magical effect upon abnormal growths. It is excellent for hardened liver and scanty flow of bile and enlarged lymphatics.

REAL SALT

Contrary to many people's belief that salt (sodium chloride) is harmful to the human body (having to do with elevated blood pressure), the truth is that not one of us can live without sodium. Sodium's presence maintains the body's electrolytic balance while enabling the body to make hydrochloric acid, the essential digestive fluid. Sodium maintains the fluidity of the blood and lymph so it doesn't become too thick. Organic sodium is found in vegetables. What we need to remember is we need organic sodium which is soluble in water. The truth is we can get all the sodium the body needs from vegetables. It is very soothing during hot weather to drink a small glass of fresh made celery juice in the morning and afternoon. This normalizes the body temperature so you are not miserable while everyone around you is perspiring heavily. It is best to not use even Realsalt with cancer. Drink celery juice every day for your organic sodium.

"Sodium is one of the important elements in the elimination of carbon dioxide from the system. Deficiency of vital organic sodium results in bronchial and lung troubles." Fresh Vegetable and Fruit Juices by N W Walker P. 42.

Salt in its natural (as opposed to processed) form first came from dried ancient sea beds. It was collected and used for flavoring and preservation. Salt's importance is cited in Scripture.

Ye are the salt of the earth: but if the salt have lost his savor, wherewith shall it be salted? It is thenceforth good for nothing, but to be cast out, and to be trodden under foot of men.[40]

About 50 years ago, the major salt producing companies in the United States began to dry salt in huge kilns at temperatures as high as 1200 degrees

---

[40]   Matthew 5:13.

Fahrenheit. While kiln-drying accelerated the production process, this drying changed salt's chemical structure by damaging it's calcium component (all salt has approximately from one half to one percent calcium by volume) from soluble, to insoluble.

The body, of course, is incapable of absorbing insoluble calcium and, therefore, results in both calcification of the inner linings of the blood vessels (hardening of the arteries) and calcium deposits in the joints (arthritis) and muscle tissue (inflammation).

Since calcium is an absolute necessary part of body chemistry, it was no coincidence that with the onset of kiln-drying, afflictions such as heart disease, arthritis, and other chemical-related diseases began to increase in this country at an alarming rate.

Today heart disease and arthritis are so prevalent in this country that even small children suffer, whereas in third-world countries such as India, China and Mexico, heart disease and arthritis are rare. This is, in part, because countries such as these do not alter their salt supply. Indeed, they can't! They do not have the machinery to do so. They eat their salt in its natural state.

Besides its effect on calcium, kiln-dried salt is also an enzyme inhibitor. Do not use white refined salt, it is an enzyme inhibitor and a poison to the body. The body needs live, vital enzymes to enable cells to synapse, or electrically communicate with one another. Become a label reader when you shop at the grocery store.

If you have a chronic condition or degenerative disease as cancer you need to eliminate all salt—even Real Salt—until you have the immune system built up again. You need to get all your sodium from vegetables such as celery or cucumbers. It takes about 2 years to totally rebuild the immune system that is why Dr. Max Gerson kept his patients on a strict program as does his daughter, Charlotte who has a clinic in Mexico. See the section on Life is in the Cells. To determine which salts are naturally prepared (or to see for yourself processed salt's insoluble nature), conduct this test on the next salt that you purchase. In fact, it would be a good idea to test all salt you use before use regardless of when or where you buy it. Mix a spoonful of salt in a glass of water and let it stand overnight. If the salt has collected on the bottom of the glass, it is insoluble; it has been processed. Salt that will not dissolve in water cannot dissolve in your body and therefore has a tendency to collect in the body organs. If it has not collected on the bottom, then it is soluble because natural salt dissolves.

Real SaltTM[41] is a brand of unprocessed, natural salt, without heating or additives, which comes directly from a huge rock salt deposit near Redmond, Utah. Since it is a natural salt, it dissolves, is not an enzyme inhibitor. Always add Real Salt after cooking your foods and not during cooking. If you cook with the RealSalt you change the good organic salt into an inorganic salt that your body can't use. As an added bonus, you need to use only one half the amount you'd normally use.

And every man that striveth for the mastery is temperate in all things. Now they do it to obtain a corruptible crown; but we an incorruptible.[42]

Some people do live without using any salt, but they do eat raw vegetables which have sodium and/or drink freshly made raw vegetable juices every day. Celery, for example, has a high percentage of sodium along with calcium. Carrot and celery juice (75 % carrot, 25 % celery) makes a great drink.

BEDSORES & SKIN GRAFTING

Bedsores can be a problem if someone is sitting in a chair or lying in bed for long periods of time. White marshmallow root in powdered form if applied dry and covered with cotton gauze or thin white cloth heals the area. Disinfect the area if you need to do that. If anyone needs skin grafting using this will restore the area without skin grafting. White marshmallow root powdered works great. You can see it doing its work of restoring the tissue. Powdered Slippery Elm is good for bedsores. It heals any raw irritated area especially internally as acid reflux, ulcers, etc.

---

[41] You may order Real Salt from Joyce Trout.
[42] I Corinthians 9:25

CASE HISTORIES

My first case history is my husband, Bud Trout:

Case history # 1:
Name: Maurice (Bud) Trout Age 59

My husband was diagnosed with prostate cancer in April of 1990. It is the third leading cause of cancer death among men. Believe me! I know how hard it is to totally rearrange your schedule to do what is necessary for a cancer patient. It is not an easy program to follow; but since it was my husband it became a labor of love. A family member needs to be totally committed to helping the relative who has cancer if they want them to get well.

They haven't the energy to do it for themselves. Bud knew the conventional treatments given by the doctor doesn't rebuild the immune system so the person has a chance to allow the body to heal itself. We have seen the results with friends & relatives who have followed the allopathic treatments. We were convinced God's way was the answer. Bud has not had any conventional treatment. He went to a natural healing doctor for blood work done periodically and an examination to see his progress but no biopsies, which are known to spread cancer.

Bud followed the raw vegetable juices, herbs, exercises with deep breathing on the rebounder, rest, detoxification, lots of green drink, good diet of fresh & raw fruits & vegetables or lightly steamed or baked, lots of flax oil, trust in our Creator, for at least one & one half to two years to totally rebuild his immune system. Bud was extremely tired, had no energy, & no color in his face for about 1 month then we started to see progress as he was able to work

for longer periods of time. We had an MRI test done in August of 1991 &
he had no sign of any cancer. Believe me, we are careful with our diet today
in 2004. Bud drinks fresh-made vegetable juice on a daily basis from our
Norwalk juicer. We eat lots of fresh & raw fruits & vegetables every day. We
thank the Lord for his healing.

The following case histories were recorded and documented in 1981 at
the Gerson Clinic in Tijuana, Mexico. I, Joyce Trout, spent a week at her
clinic in 1986 & I saw her program first hand.

Case History #2:
Name: John Doe Age: 61

Prostate Cancer & kidney polyps On full disability because he had 3
herniated discs. Discs pressing on the sciatic nerve. Constant pain. His left
thigh had gone down by 50 % atrophy. He had high blood pressure. Went to
Gerson Clinic because of the cancer. From the first day he never had another
kidney polyp because kidney polyps are animal related and Gerson Clinic
never serves meat or meat-related products. Two years later he went back to
the original doctor, who was the head of the Oncology at the University of
California in Santa Barbara and was examined. X-ray of the spine showed
normal spine, discs rebuilt, no cancer, his thigh 93% rebuilt. Mrs Gerson
asked the patient on the phone, "Did they take your disability payments away
since you have healed so beautifully?" Patient said, "No, They didn't believe
me". He is still alive and well in 1992.

Case History #3
Name: Debbie Spears Age: 27

Melanoma tumor on her arm. Doctor cut out tumor-deep excision.
Doctor told her they got all of the cancer. Six months later had another
cancer under her arm. Doctor wanted to cut it out. Patient refused. Went to
Gerson Clinic.

One month later after Gerson treatment, melanoma tumor disappeared.
Patient is alive and well in 1992.

Case History #4
Name: Melva Blackburn Age 66

Constant medical problems beginning in 1940. Started with kidney disease and many operations. Constant treatment until 1979. Heart & coronary artery disease. Whiplash in 1964 did not respond to treatment. Diabetes: on medication since 1965. Poor control (neuropathy) of legs & feet. Cushing's syndrome (adrenal gland disease-overweight, fatigue, weakness, osteoporosis, edema, susceptibility to infection. Pneumonia at least twice a year since 1964, enlarged liver, arthritis in all bones including ears, anxiety, ataxia, confusion, Alzheimer's disease (premature old age, senility). Years on drugs & many surgeries. Started Gerson therapy Oct. 1979 & feels fine now. Astounded all doctors who examined her later and confirmed her good health. Comment: Numerous "incurable" diseases-kidney disease, heart disease, adrenal disease (cushing's syndrome), diabetes, osteoporosis, arthritis, Alzheimer's disease-cured by Gerson Therapy.

Case history # 5
Name: Irmgard Ament Age: 56

In March 1975, biopsy showed invasive type squamous cell carcinoma of cervix. Had surgical conization of cervix followed by cobalt treatment & radium implants for an almost unbelievable 13,065 rads. The result was severe burns and damage to the transverse colon, rectum, and vagina with progressive weakness and anemia. Her doctors gave a hopeless prognosis. Began Gerson Therapy in 1976 with improper juicer and non organic vegetables. Had some success but not enough. Lung cancer diagnosed in husband in 1977 he accepted allopathic treatment such as radiation & chemo. & died in 1979. In 1977 she got proper juicer and began strict Gerson Therapy. Her energy, strength, and well-being improved but her cancer returned when she went off the Gerson Therapy too soon in order to help her husband with his illness. She went back on the Gerson Therapy in 1979 after her husband died & the cancer disappeared. In January 1980 after her checkup her oncologist said, "There was very good healing in her body". He found no cancer, no burns, no adhesions & no scars. He was puzzled.

Comment: Hopeless cancer and severe burns from excessive radiation cured by Gerson Therapy. It is very important to remember that all above mentioned case histories except my husband were interviews that took place in 1981 & in 1992 all former patients at the Gerson Clinic were alive & well. My husband, Bud Trout is alive & well as of this writing in 2008 after home treatment based on the Gerson Therapy with some other treatments of my own.

Case History # 6
Name: Jaquie Davison (This case history is Jaquie's personal testimony (with Jane Storm) was taken from her book, Cancer Winner).

August 1974: I was 36 years old when cancer crept in like a thief in the night & I found myself face to face with my mortality. There was a golf ball size tumor in my right groin and smaller ones in my diaphragm area, left arm & left leg below the knee. Diagnosis:

(Scripps Memorial Hospital Lab) Malignant Melanoma-toenail tissue in lymph nodes and soft tissue. It was too far advanced for me to get much help from allopathic medicine. I sought the natural health route and found the field most confusing with various therapies that conflict greatly. I found myself floundering as the disease progressed.

Dec. 1974: Started a 30 day fast.(I don't recommend a fast as you need to be under the care of a natural healing doctor) Lasted only 10 days (holidays) Passed two large polyps with enemas. No progression of disease at that time. January 1975: Went to see Dr. Hugh Carruthers in Ariz. Rigid tests showed body seriously deteriorated. Went to a naturopath in Calif. He treated with extensive vitamin therapy-one month no change. He said," I can't help you".

March 1975: Losing all faith as disease progresses rapidly. New tumors appearing all the time, desperate. Tried to fast again but it lasted only five days. Liver spots on face & shoulder. Moles appearing all over my body & stomach bloating. Bloated 30 pounds in 2 months. Tumors in neck & head. I have so many I have lost count of them.

June 1975: Told Ron (my husband has moved mountains for me) "If my body pathology doesn't change soon I am going to die". I began giving away personal items among my daughters (I've taken them back since I got well) My husband read Ann Wigmore's book called Why Suffer? I remembered my mother sprouting wheat grass years ago & while she was doing the wheat grass juice she had a blood test and the doctor told her she had the purest blood he had ever seen. I started sprouting wheat & my stamina was increased when I drank the juice. There was no significant change in my physical condition as I needed something more. I had friends all over praying for me. Some churches devoted entire days to pray for me. As the cards & letters came in my son, Ralphie (12 years old) said, "God won't disappoint all these people". He was right! God's amazing grace touched my body & soul. I remind my children daily that my healing was not an accident but a miracle of God. Jane Storm: You heard me & brought the book to me, "Has Dr Max Gerson a True Cancer Cure?' It was the information I had been searching for. Because of you, Jane Storm, I have held my two new grand babies (born in September of 1975) in my arms with joy unspeakable, because I did not think I'd ever see them. God graced my life for some purpose. Perhaps it was for me to pass a ray of hope along to the children who will suffer with cancer. By doing so, I am saying Thank you, Jane!

I sent for the book, A Cancer Therapy also by Dr. Max Gerson and then told Ron of Dr. Gerson's emphasis on the right juicer. It is a very expensive machine. I also read aloud to Ron from the book I found at the health food store called Fresh Vegetable & Fruit Juices by N W Walker. The juices have to be ground & pressed. I used carrot juice made on a centrifugal machine for 6 months with no noticeable results.

Just 5 days on the Norwalk juicer & I saw remarkable results. When the centrifugal machine came out, Dr. Gerson was excited believing that the therapy would be simplified. He found that he did not get the same good results. A physicist told him that there is a positive electricity in the center of the centrifugal machine that negates the negative (potassium) juice.

Tuesday" Ron came home with the Norwalk juicer and a bag of carrots. I got the apples, beets, sprouts, and wheat grass and started to make juice. I had to make a fresh one each hour and take coffee enemas every four hours to stimulate the bile ducts to dump & cleanse the liver so in turn the liver would be able to cleanse the blood.

Saturday: I cannot sleep. My body is numb and tingly in parts. It feels as if the life is leaving it. When I doze, I hallucinate. I told Ron, "Maybe if I eat something I am not supposed to, this action will stop. I can't stand the cure. I read the section in the book on reaction and inflammation over and over and now I know this action is necessary for the healing.

Sunday: Noon, I passed a tumor from my colon. The cells were plump and black like tiny watermelon seeds. There was a severe pain where the tumor pulled loose and the discharge was so acid or hot, that it scalded me terribly. Half-conscious and bleeding, I was scared. Ron wanted to take me to the hospital but I refused. "I just can't believe that food is going to kill me". My colon bled for 3 days. There was a constant inflammation in the area where it pulled loose for 2 months. By 6 P M I was telling friends, "I'm not going to die, God has delivered me". I felt wonderful. No sleep again that night as I had to do juices and enemas.

Monday: Still no sleep. Body demands constant tending or I feel myself slipping into a coma.

Tuesday: I slept 4 hours in the evening when awakened in an extremely high fever. The sweat was falling in big drops and my body was rosy all over. The soles of my feet were greatly inflamed. Ipraised God again, for my body was producing its own immunity (asDr. Gerson promised) to the cancer cells all over my body. Reactions: I found that I did not experience one reaction that was not explained in the book. I spent hours of coffee enema time studying A Cancer Therapy by Dr. Max Gerson until the covers fell off. The Late Dr. Gerson was German, but I am so proud he walked America, too. A journalist, Mr. Haught, who wrote Has Dr. Max Gerson a True Cancer Cure, was sent out to expose Dr. Gerson as a fraud. He gained a great respect for the doctor & asked, "Where are the monuments to this great man?" God willing I'd like to be a part of that monument building, by telling his story and mine at every opportunity. I want to publicly thank my daughter, Regina Rose, 14 years old, for leaving school this year to devote her time to caring for me and running our household. She nursed me through some times when neither of us thought I'd live to see the next day. No one has ever known a more loving "Angel of Mercy". Thank you, My Precious Daughter.

Dead Cells: As my feet began feeling better, I noticed an amazing thing. The lymph was emptying out of the pores of the soles of my feet and ridding the body of black debris. Also, my right underarm turned almost black and I could see the cells under the skin gradually diminishing in size until they were completely dissolved. I had the pigment from my feet analyzed and the lab verified that it was melanin pigment containing keratin. It pours out of my body like coal soot. My surgeon (I found no doctor familiar with the therapy to help me so I've been on my own) said he had heard of such a thing, vaguely, but he never dreamed he would ever be this close to a case.

Two Months After Therapy: I had the large tumor (the size of a lemon by now) removed surgically. It was on my artery and broke open on the doctor. The substance was gushy. He exclaimed, "I've never seen anything like this before! It looks like an open pit mine in here". The cells were dead and a lymph node in the covering of the tumor contained dead melanoma cells, also.

My Pharmacist said, "I know enough about melanoma to know that when a tumor is removed with dead cells, something beyond our understanding is taking place." Seven Months Later, March 1976: The debris is still flowing out my pores. It is exciting to see the dead cells leaving my body. Because my body was poisoned from head to toe and the dead cells are almost metallic, it may be a year before I am completely clean. When a tumor turns loose, I get very very sick. My heart beats fast. There is a tremendous pressure in my head and I feel tingly and numb. I take the juices and enemas (more than scheduled) until it passes. Many times the dead cells (resembling coal soot) pass out my colon encapsulated in mucus and look like an eel. As soon as it passed I have a buoyant feeling of relief. The time consumed may be from 30 minutes to 2 hrs. My Physical Condition Now? I'm healthier than I have been in years & healthier than most people. Friends say that in these 7 months I have lost 20 years off my age. (I did look pretty bad at "Death's Door") My weekly migraine headaches left when I passed the tumor from my colon. The numbness in my neck and head is gone. The yellow skin and film over my eyes is gone. I'm in the pink now! My hair is growing fast and abundantly. It had diminished to almost nothing. My menstrual cycle is a perfect 28 days. The liver spots on my face and shoulder are almost gone. My ears were dry and the wax is normal now. Even that was exciting.

The edema all over my body left when I went off salt (cancer cells love a sodium condition). I have abundant energy and I jog and do yoga exercises for an hour a day. If I were not on such a rigid schedule, I could do a day's work as well as anyone. Before the therapy, I would catch cold often and almost die. I would sleep day and night. Now I sleep 6 or 7 hours a night and have no need for naps. My chronic skin problem and scalp eczema are gone. My skin is satin smooth. Many tumors are gone already. I've had new ones since the therapy and that was right after surgery. They went away overnight. Right now I have tremendous action going on in my neck and head and the black debris is working its way out my mouth and tongue. Doesn't that sound like science fiction! It has been a most exciting experience for me. I cut my knuckle off and had a big hole. In ten days I had a perfect new knuckle, no scar! I also had a serious burn. In seven days you couldn't tell I had been burned. It healed perfectly.

I HAD A TOOTH MEND ITSELF! During an inflammation I found myself rubbing a tooth that had a cavity. I had delayed having it fixed because I was trying to detoxify my body. A large chunk came off the tooth and I was upset knowing I'd have to rush to the dentist. I finally got the nerve to examine the damage. The tooth was covered with new enamel. It was yellow and sensitive for about 10 days, but now it is as sound as it can be. I read once that mung bean sprouts would rebuild teeth. I use a lot of them in my juices. I was so excited that I got out Gerson's book and began reading case histories again. One woman with bone cancer had pins in her legs. The bone grew back and bent the pins! (He shows x-rays of the case). A colostomy grew back entirely normal!

What's a little tooth enamel! Wow! With God all things are possible. Where are the monuments? Dr Gerson says this is not solely a cancer therapy, but it is to restore the liver so the body can defend itself against all diseases. There is an appendix to the book giving a less rigid program that everyone can follow for the ultimate health.

IF THIS THERAPY CAN CURE THE CANCER (MOST POISONED BODY OF ALL) PATIENT, JUST IMAGINE WHAT IT CAN DO FOR THE MERELY SICK OR RUNDOWN! SOMETHING EXCITING HAPPENS WHEN WE GIVE OUR BODIES LIVE OXYGEN AND ENZYMES AS GOD INTENDED US TO. EVERY PART OF THE BODY HAS COME ALIVE AND WANTS TO MOVE!

LOCATION OF BOOKS, PRODUCTS & PLACES

You may purchase Dr. Christopher's products (such as BFC (Regeneration) and Red Clover Combination Teas and Salves), video cassettes, audio cassette tapes and books, and products such as the Green Star juicers, etc. from Joyce Trout, 175 Music Barn Lane, Monterey, TN 38574. Call 931-498-2844. You may write to me whichever is most convenient.

The Herbal Home Health Care & the School of Natural Healing books by Dr. John R. Christopher N.D., M.H. are also available from Joyce.

SUPPLEMENTAL MATERIAL

Remember your immune system is what destroys the cancer. You need to have a strong immune system to do that so you have to rebuild the immune system with raw vegetable & fresh made fruit juices, raw foods, herbal teas that detoxify the whole body such as Dr. John Christopher's Red Clover Combination tea, Miracle 2 products that alkalinize the system which is very acidic now. They also open up our billions of pores (so the poisons can come out through the skin) when you soak in the tub for 45 minutes to one hour with one ounce of the soap & one ounce of the neutralizer. You need to follow God's Plan of eating fruits, vegetables, whole grains, seeds, and nuts (almonds) with much fresh and raw (80%, if possible).

Garlic is an excellent food that rebuilds the immune system plus it gets rid of any infection in the body. It cleanses the arteries and blood vessels. It is antiseptic and it destroys the bad bacteria. You can use it in cooking or peel the cloves and put in the blender with water and blend well and drink 2-3 ounces. Garlic stimulates the gastric juices and corrects putrefactive and gaseous conditions in the stomach. It arrests intestinal putrefaction and infection while stimulating the healthful growth of the friendly bacteria. Cancer is a fermentative disease that feeds on poisons such as the undigested protein which feeds the cancer. Garlic helps to destroy tumors as well. Remember to take an all plant enzymes digest aid with each meal so you can break down the proteins and fats properly so the undigested proteins aren't feeding the cancer cells & causing them to grow more.

IRON DRINK

This raises the blood platelet count. It helps the body to use oxygen properly because the iron carries the oxygen molecule. It will help anemia & other blood iron related problems. It is great for a cancer patient as their body doesn't use iron properly. Liquid natural products such as iron drink, juices, & herb teas are absorbed readily.

1 gallon of grape juice
1 cup of raisins-organic if possible & unsulphured
½-1 cup dried dark apricots-unsulphured
½-1 cup Black strap Molasses

Let it soak over night & the next morning put it in the refrigerator.

Drink 4 ounces 4 times a day till you have your blood count back to normal. Listen to your body & see what works for you. You may want to cut the recipe in half. You may eat the fruit, also.

Foods rich in iron are raisins, apricots, strawberries, watermelon, grape juice, spinach, red beets, black strap molasses, tomatoes, asparagus, figs, plums, grapes, prunes, celery, seeds, turnips, celery, looseleaf lettuce, & wheat germ. Some herb teas that contain iron are Comfrey, Yellow Dock is the richest in iron, Red Clover, Fennel, Elderberry, Pau d'arco tea, Parsley, & Dandelion. Parsley tea cleanses the kidneys & urinary tract. This is only a partial list do your own research to find more. Don't take iron tablets if you are low in iron as they can cause duodenal ulcers because they stay in the duodenum for a period of time before they dissolve. God's Plan works if you work the Plan. I have used this with women that were hemorrhaging & it restored their blood count to normal in a matter of days and it has restored the iron needed by cancer patients.

When we do all on our part to have health, them may we expect that the blessed results will follow and we can ask God in faith to bless our efforts for the preservation of health. He will then answer our prayer if His name can be glorified thereby. But let all understand that they have a work to do. God will not work in a miraculous manner to preserve the health of persons who are taking a sure course to make themselves sick, by their careless inattention to the laws of health. Counsels on Diet & Foods P. 26 by E. G. White

CANCER OUTLINE

You will find that if you eat 80-85% fresh & raw fruits & vegetables along with the program outlined in my Cancer book you will get well faster and feel much better. God has given us a healing mechanism so the body always tends toward wellness but it is up to us to feed the body the right nutrients which are rich in potassium so the immune system can work well so it can heal the body.

The Miracle 2 will speed your recovery. They are 100% natural & they will pull our toxins & even inorganic metals. When you have Cancer it isn't good to be cleaning your house with chemicals as they further weaken the immune system & breathing them isn't good for the lungs plus you absorb the chemicals through your skin as you are doing the cleaning. You can replace every chemical in your house with the Miracle 2 products. Take the neutralizer internally as it alkalinizes the system. Cancer patients are getting good results with 4 to 6 ounces of it every day. Remember you need 20 to 30 bitter apricot seeds a day. Take about 5 or 6 at a time throughout the day. They contain B17 or laetrile to kill the cancer cells. 5 to 7 tablespoons of Barlean's flax oil a day is important as it oxygenates the system & destroys cancer cells or tumors. Eat only fruits, vegs., whole grains, seeds, & nuts. Take a digest aid with each meal as your body isn't breaking down the proteins & fats properly so the undigested protein feeds the cancer cells. A digest aid helps to break down the foods. You can buy whole papaya & eat some fresh papaya after meals as that is a good digest aid.

Rebuilding the immune system means eating God's diet, trust in God for healing, detoxifying the body, lots of raw vegetable juices, exercise, moving the lymphatic system with the minitrampoline, & a positive mental attitude (remember God's promises are true).

Gen. 1:29 God says, "Behold I have given you every herb bearing seed, which is upon the face of the earth & every tree, in the which is the fruit of a tree yielding seed, to you it shall be for meat."

Ps. 104:14 God tells us, "I have given the grass for the cattle & the herbs for the service of man". God is the Great Physician.

CANOLA OIL

Olive oil comes from olives, peanut oil from peanuts, sunflower oil from sunflowers but what is a canola? Canola is not the name of a natural plant but a made-up name from the words Canada & oil. Canola is a genetically engineered plant developed from the Rapeseed plant, which is part of the mustard family of plants. According to AgriAlternatives these Rapeseed oils have long been used to produce oils for purposes that are toxic to humans & other animals. The Canadian Government & industry paid our Federal Food & Drug Administration (FDA) $50 million dollars to have canola oil placed on the (GRAS) list "Generally Recognized As Safe. Thus a new industry was created. Laws were enacted affecting international trade, commerce, & traditional diets. Studies with animals were disastrous. Rats developed fatty degeneration of heart, kidneys, adrenals, & thyroid gland. When they stopped giving them canola oil the deposits dissolved but scar tissue remained on all vital organs. No studies on humans were made before money was spent to promote canola oil in the USA.

Rapeseed oil is poisonous to living things & is an excellent insect repellent being used to kill aphids for years. It is very effective as it suffocates them. The oil is used as a lubricant, fuel, soap, & synthetic rubber base & to illuminate for color pages in magazines. It is an industrial oil not for human use. It is not a food.

Rape oil (Canola Oil) is strongly related to symptoms of emphysema, respiratory disturbances, anemia, constipation, irritability, & blindness in animals & humans. Canola Oil is genetically engineered rapeseed. Canada paid the FDA $50 million to have the rapeseed registered as "safe". Source: Young Again magazine & other sources. Rapeseed is a lubricating oil used by small industry. It has never been tested for human consumption. It is considered a toxic poison which when processed becomes rancid very quickly. This should tell you something the insects won't eat it. The Rapeseed has been shown to cause lung cancer. Wall Street Journal-June 7, 1995 some possible side effects include loss of vision, disruption of the nervous system, respiratory illness, anemia, heart disease, cancer, low birth weights in infants, & irritability in adults. Rapeseed has a cumulative effect, taking almost 10 years to manifest itself. It inhibits proper metabolism of foods a normal enzyme function. Canola is a trans fatty acid (c22) & this makes it hydrogenated. Canola oil contains a long chain fatty acid called erucic acid, which is irritating to mucus membranes. The buildup of long-chain fatty acids destroys the myelin or protective sheath on the nerve cells. Canola oil is a long chain fatty acid that has been treated to very high temperatures 300 degrees. Avoid all of the hydrogenated oils as they are deposited on the arteries & blood vessels to cause hardening of the arteries, high blood pressure,. strokes, heart disease, etc

Peanut oil & other oils are being replaced with Canola oil. It is in many processed foods such as peanut butter. The reason being it is the cheapest oil & the Canadian Government subsidizes it to industries involved in food processing. We have other choices for oils such as Olive oil or Flax oil which destroys tumor tissue & oxygenates the system. The flax oil taken on a daily basis lowers high blood pressure, high triglycerides, & high cholesterol if you watch your diet & don't eat meat & dairy products which are too high in protein & fat. A man worked as a quality control taster at an apple chip factory where canola oil was used for frying & he developed numerous health problems loose teeth, gum disease, gum & nail beds turned gray, numb hands & feet with cramps, swollen arms & legs upon arising in the AM, extreme joint pain especially in hands, cloudy vision, constipation with stools like black marbles, hearing loss, skin tears if bumped, lack of energy, hair loss, & heart pains. He quit 5 years ago

& still has some joint pain, gum disease, & numbness. A fellow worker about 30 years old who ate very little of the products had a routine check up & found his blood vessels were like those of an eighty year old man. Why do they foist such products on the public because it is all about money? It is also a very cheap oil to produce. The government subsidies Canola oil to some industries involved in food processing, bakeries, & schools. Don't be fooled into using canola oil as it is not fit for human consumption it can harm you.

Even after the processing it is a penetrating oil. It turns rancid very fast so now you have many free radicals to cause more health problems. It emits cancer causing chemicals. Materials taken from a Report by Tom Valentine called Canola Oil Report & FATS THAT HEAL & FATS THAT KILL BY UDO ERASMUS.

Canola oil was widely used in animal feed in England & Europe between 1986 & 1991 when it was thrown out. Remember the "Mad Cow Disease" scare, when millions of unfortunate cattle were slaughtered in the UK so they wouldn't infect people. Cattle were being fed a mixture containing material from dead sheep & sheep suffer from a disease called "scrapie". They had canola oil in the feed, remember. It was thought this was how the "Mad Cow" began to infiltrate the human chain. What is interesting is when Canola oil was removed from animal feed "scrapie" disappeared.

COTTONSEED OIL

Has anyone ever heard of cotton being a food? I haven't heard of it. Peanut oil comes from peanuts & Olive oil comes from olives & Flax oil comes from the flax plant. Now think where does cottonseed oil come from? Of course it comes from the deadly cotton plant. Is cotton a food? Why then is it put in our foods? Read the labels & you will find it in many potato chips & other processed foods. It is used because it is a cheap oil. I read labels & I will not buy anything that has cottonseed oil or canola oil in them as they are very harmful to our bodies. See my information on Canola oil for the health problems it causes. Once you start reading labels you will be amazed at all the food items that have Cottonseed oil in them.

Cotton: The Deadliest Textile By Judy Yablonski, at AlterNet.org Aug. 15, 2002 may give you more information. Cottonseed oil is used in common snack foods, such as potato chips & cookies plus other prepared foods, as well. The main problem is the oil extracted from the cotton is full of toxic pesticides & fertilizers & it is genetically engineered. The dairy cows accumulate pesticide residues in their tissues so if you are drinking milk you get the pesticides, too. Cotton is a textile not a food so they are not well regulated. The cotton growers use chemicals regularly that have been banned from food crops because they are highly toxic. The cotton industry consumes 10 % of the world's pesticides & 25% of the insecticides according to the Pesticide Action Network (PAN).

Oils were not made to cook with as this makes them harmful to the body. The oils are then deposited on the arteries & blood vessels to cause high blood pressure, high cholesterol, high triglycerides, strokes, heart attacks, & etc. Cottonseed oil contains transfatty acids which are very harmful to the body. See the Report on Canola oil for more on trans fatty acids. You want essential fatty acids as in organic flax oil or olive oil. These nourish & feed every organ, destroy tumor tissue, oxygenate the system & etc.

CAFFEINE

Caffeine is converted to uric acid in the system which causes gout, arthritis, & much more. Then the Caffeine interferes with the laboratory determination of the uric acid level in the blood & may cause a missed diagnosis of gout because you get a low reading of uric acid. We have a blood brain barrier to protect the brain from harmful chemicals but this harmful chemical called

Caffeine sneaks past the blood brain barrier to stimulate the brain cortex where thoughts are made & the brain medulla where body functions are regulated.

The immediate effects begin shortly after taking the coffee or soda containing the Caffeine. They last about 4 hours. Caffeine may cause racing of the heart, imperfect balance, high pitched or abnormal pitch of the voice.

Insomnia, racing but disconnected thoughts, headache, vertigo, restless legs, agitation, irritability, general discomfort, poor memory, fatigue, finger tremor, depression occurs so you need another cup to keep you on a high. The list goes on & on. Every type of disease has been attributed to Caffeine. If you drink Caffeine drinks you are on a Titanic course with a diabolical iceberg. You unfortunately won't win.

When you take hot chocolate, regular tea such as Lipton, sodas like Coca Cola, Sprite, or coffee, which all contain Caffeine & other harmful chemicals, the entire small bowel is able to absorb this energy-producing substance called cyclic AMP 1200% more effectively. You say "Great" but it isn't as it is like putting mothballs in your gas tank with your gasoline. You may have a lot more energy for a little while but you will soon burn out the engine.

Caffeine is a mind affecting drug classified with alcohol & nicotine. Some people think they are doing themselves a favor by drinking decaffeinated coffee but trust me you are not any better off than you are drinking the regular coffee. The process they use is worse than the caffeine they are trying to eliminate and you still have some caffeine in the coffee. Do some research for yourself. Caffeine is rapidly & completely absorbed from the gastrointestinal tract & passes through the central nervous system. It lasts 3 & ½-4 hours. Drugs are stored in the liver so you have to detoxify the liver plus the whole body to cleanse the body of the effects of the Caffeine after you stop drinking the Caffeine drinks. You get a high with the Caffeine & then a letdown as the Caffeine blocks the energy productions in the body. Now you have nutrient imbalance, risk of blood clotting, thinning of bones, nervous fatigue, & depression. Caffeine causes constriction of the arteries, which is not to your benefit, it increases the load on the heart by speeding up the rate & it can raise blood pressure & it reduces the heart's own blood supply making it labor more. It interferes with the function of the renal tubules. Sodas & other Caffeine drinks dehydrate the body (they pull out the water). This causes all kinds of problems because we are 75% water & all the organs need water to perform their processes. The skin dries out as well & your skin can't breathe & eliminate the toxins like it should. Take the digestion. The digestive tract needs water to digest your food. To help this process, so it doesn't pull water from somewhere else in the body where it is needed, it is best to drink a full glass of water about 20 minutes before you eat. Squeeze a half lemon in the water. Lemons alkalinize the body & help get rid of the acidity. They are antiseptic, too. The lemon is a wonderful stimulant to the liver, liquefies the bile, cleanses the system of impurities. Lemons are rich in potassium so they repair the damage to the nerve cells & brain that the Caffeine has caused. It is also rich in calcium & magnesium so its calcium is absorbed & put to use to make healthy bones. Lemons are great for colds, coughs, sore throat, flu, asthma, heart burn, liver problems, etc. We start the day with a fresh squeezed lemon in a glass of very warm water. It gets everything going in the body. For more on the benefits of the lemon see Back to Eden P. 658-661

Chocolate is as harmful as the caffeine as it may contain 112 mgs. per cup of cocoa. It also contains tannin which has caused cancers of the digestive tract. Cocoa ties up calcium & other nutrients you may get from wonderful sources as vegetables, whole grains, legumes, & greens. Chocolate interferes with calcium absorption. Theobromine in the chocolate causes abnormal gland growth, central nervous system stimulation, sleeplessness, depression, if the kidneys don't work well the theobromine accumulates to high blood levels. It has recently been said to cause enlargement of the prostate. Chocolate is very bitter by itself so huge amounts of sugar are added to make it taste good. Sugar interferes with calcium absorption & destroys the white blood cells which destroy germs, it makes it hard to concentrate, promotes tooth decay, & peptic ulcers. They also add milk to it to help eliminate the unpleasant taste of the cocoa this causes fermentation, slow digestion, causes the red blood cells to cluster together in groups, blocks capillary circulation in the brain & causes poor mental performance.

Cacao beans are grown in pods each pod containing 20-30 beans. One pod may give you 1-2 ounces of dry beans. The seeds are bitter & astringent, white, very pale purple or deep purple. The chocolate is made from the bitter seeds. Pods are cut down, the beans are scooped out & now they ferment for 3-8 days at temperatures up to 140 degrees. The fermentation is done in boxes, on mats, or in wicker bags. This helps develop the chocolate. This takes place in the yards of the local farmer. Children & adults walk over the piles, insects, rodents, small animals & other living creatures make their nests in the piles & other contamination occurs. Cacao beans have a lot of aflatoxins (cancer causing substance gotten from mold because they mold during the process). Aflatoxins are the most potent cancer producing agents. After they ferment the seeds are sun or kiln dried & shipped to the manufacturers of the chocolate. There is much more in the manufacture but space doesn't allow me to write it all. There is a booklet published by the U.S. Dept. Of Health, Education & Welfare entitled "The Food Defect Action Levels" that lists the current levels for natural or unavoidable defects in food. In chocolate it lists the natural defects in the form of "insect, rodent, & other allowable natural contaminants" that the FDA allows. Chocolate & chocolate liquor in the manufacture of such products as Hershey's chocolate are up to 120 insect fragments per 8 oz. or two rodent hair & 16 insect parts & they still carry the blessing of the FDA. When I read this I am thankful for Carob which is a wonderful substitute for chocolate.

Case History: An 11 year old boy had severe abdominal pain & he was vomiting blood. He very suddenly developed tiny spots of hemorrhage in his skin all over his body. He was hospitalized & they discovered his attacks were brought on in a few minutes by eating chocolate. Chocolate is the common cause of "pruritus ani" an uncomfortable itch around the anus, the terminal part of the rectum.

When you give up chocolate this condition stops. Caffeine is not a friend. If you have a problem with Caffeine in any form give it to the Lord He is the only one who can help you *get over the addiction.* God is able & willing to help us in any situation.

HYPOGLYCEMIA/DIABETES

This is #2 in a series entitled: THE GOOD NEWS YOU SHOULD KNOW! There are 4 books as follows: Cancer, Degeneration of the Bone, Strokes, And Hypoglycemia/Diabetes. This book tells you how to regulate the blood sugar with herbs, how to get the lymphatic system working at top efficency so the poisons can be gotten out of the body, how to restore the Pancreas to normal function & much more. God has given us the tools we need to get the body to restore itself. I tell you how to rebuild the immune system so it can allow the body to heal itself. What can you do if the kidneys shutdown? Do you need to go on kidney dialysis? No, God has a program for you. There are several testimonials such as the young man of 21 who had only 60% vision, severe kidney damage, doctors said he needed a kidney transplant. He had severe bladder problems. The doctors wanted to remove his bladder and give him a bag. His whole body was swollen with edema and his blood pressure was very high. Two weeks on a complete program at the Gerson Clinic and he was feeling so much better. In 6 weeks he was almost totally back to being a healthy young man again. You'll want to read his entire story. You will need a step by step program to follow. What can you do if someone has a gangrenous foot? Everything is outlined telling you what to do so the foot can return to normal. God has given us the blueprint to follow so the body can heal itself. There is a very simple herbal remedy for kidney infection that may surprise you. It works every time. Essential fatty acids help to dissolve adipose tissue, & permit good weight control. They also lower cholesterol, triglycerides, & high blood pressure with the proper diet. How about putting the myelin sheath back on the nerve cells as in multiple sclerosis. You'll find many pages of its benefits for all degenerative diseases. I've given you enough about the book on Hypoglycemia/Diabetes if this doesn't convince you of the importance of this book for your family & friends nothing more I could say will convince you.

I am looking for Medical Missionaries to share my books with others so feel free to call.

LEUKEMIA

This is a disease that is manifested by excessively rapid increase of the white blood cells, causing the breakdown of red blood cells. The tissue of the spleen may enlarge, other lymphatic glands, too, plus the bone marrow. The disease is attended with increasing exhaustion. There may be internal hemorrhage as in the retina of the eye. It is caused by insufficient organic atoms in the diet. This means you are not getting enough live enzymes which are found in the fruits, vegetables, sprouts, juices, and herbs. Leukemia is caused by too much cooked food, starches, sweets, meats, dairy products, health foods such as frichik, and processed foods. You need to strengthen the immune system & the lymphocytes which fight viral infection. Cleanse the blood by detoxifying the whole body, and then begin to rebuild it. Leukemia is known as cancer of the blood.

Anemia results from the crowding out of normal bone marrow cells, preventing normal production of red blood cells and platelets. There is often uncontrolled infection owing to lack of mature or normal white blood cells. Carbon dioxide & other waste gases are being reabsorbed into the life-giving oxygen in the body & this causes the anemia because the iron is not getting to the cells. When the body doesn't have enough oxygen one atom of oxygen unites with carbon to form carbon monoxide. The body doesn't have enough iron in the blood to carry enough oxygen to the cells so they can breathe & throw off their wastes. The cells die & new cells are not produced fast enough to replace the decaying & dead cells. Pus is formed when the cells decay. You need to have lots of oxygen in the blood to carry away the waste. Apples have the most oxygen of all the fruits (winesap are the best). God has put iron & oxygen in almost all the fruits & vegetables we eat but we must eat them raw. The principal source of organic iron & oxygen is fresh fruit. Beets, turnips, tomatoes, spinach, looseleaf lettuce, cabbage, celery, carrots, spinach, parsley, squash, mustard greens, dandelion, & watercress are a few of the vegetables rich in iron. We need lots of fresh air, exercise, rest, excellent water or right now for Leukemia the distilled water of the vegetables in the form of fresh juice. Muscular movement & exercise get the lymphatic system going so walk & deep breathe. Comfrey & Alfalfa contain Vitamin B12. Dandelion is rich in potassium, iron, & nutritive salts which purify the blood & destroy the acids in the blood & allow healing to take place. Sprouts are an excellent way of getting enough of your nutrients because you increase the vitamin content by 500%. You can sprout any seeds but I like lentils & alfalfa.

I would follow the basic program as outlined in my Cancer book. It gives a full program to follow to rebuild the immune system by detoxifying the body. For Acute Leukemia I would go on a 100% fresh & raw diet with your raw vegetable juices plus green drink.

Remember the carrot juice molecule is analogous to the blood molecule. The raw vegetable juices bypass the digestive tract & in 10-15 minutes carry the iron, oxygen, & potassium to the cells so healing can begin. You can have a healing reaction when you go on a 100% raw diet so listen to your body if it is too intense eat something cooked as a baked potato with flaxseed oil on it. The cooked food slows down the cleansing process. I would find a Natural Healing doctor to monitor my progress as I improve my diet. I have a list of them by states if you need one. Read Life is in the Cells in my Cancer book for more details. A good juice combination is carrot, red beet, dandelion, & spinach. Dr. N. W. Walker wrote a book called Fresh Vegetable & Fruit Juices. It tells you the minerals that are in each juice & you can find what is the best juice combination for your disease. You need at least 2 quarts of vegetable juice a day. 3 qts of juice is much better.

Dry skin brush before your bath to get the lymph flowing. 60% of our elimination is through our skin. I would recommend a nylon back brush for brushing the skin. Remember to start brushing the hands and go in a circular motion. Always work toward the heart. It takes about three minutes of your time before your daily bath. Never use harsh soap on the skin as this destroys the good flora or the acid mantle layer we have on our skin to help fight infection. Harsh soaps, also, clog the pores. When you block up the pores you force the poisons back into the lymph system and this will cause worse problems some where else in the body. Miracle 2 is the best soap for batheing & shampoo as it opens the pores so the skin breathes.

Cleanse the colon as per the colon section in my Cancer booklet. FenLB is an excellent colon cleanser. You must have an easy elimination for every meal you eat. We all have a coating of fecal matter on the walls of the colon. The FenLB loosens these deposits and allows the body to absorb the nutrients from your food. The FenLB gets the peristaltic motion going, also. See my paper on

FenLB for more information. Most people only absorb 10-15% of their nutrients because of the fecal lining on the walls of the intestinal tract. You need lots of the friendly bacteria. This helps the peristaltic motion in the colon, also. They protect you from harmful bacteria, yeast infection, viruses, & they counteract the cancer-causing compounds in the colon. We have many strains of friendly bacteria on the mucus membrane of the intestinal tract. Flora Source contains 14 different strains of the friendly bacteria. It should be at your health food store.

Read the section on the liver in the Cancer booklet. The whole body is involved when you have a disease so you have to reactivate it. Every cancer patient has liver problems so take the liver herbs & rub the liver and colon areas with olive oil 5 minutes before applying castor oil.

Make sure you are taking a digest aid with each meal. I am a distributor for an excellent one called Digest. The body isn't breaking down the proteins and fats properly so they are causing mucus and poisons in the system to further clog the bloodstream. It has all plant enzymes to digest everything we might eat so the body can use the food to form good blood cells. When the body doesn't digest the proteins properly they float around in the bloodstream and the cancer cells latch onto them and form more cancer cells. The cancer cell has a protein coating on it. Cancer cells love undigested protein. A digest aid is a must if you want to get well. Use raw almonds as they have Vitamin B17 as do all the pits of the fruits.

You need to cleanse the cells so the blood can be cleansed. Dr. Christopher has an herbal combination which is his cancer formulation for cleansing the bloodstream. It is his Red Clover combination. It contains herbs which will cleanse each cell in the body. This tea cleanses the liver, lymphatics, bloodstream, cells, kidneys, and helps the colon, too. This combination is necessary for total healing.

I would drink several glasses of green drink every day. This acts like a blood transfusion to the body. Start with the best water in the blender. In the Spring you can pick fresh Plantain, Chickweed, Comfrey, Parsley, Dandelion or Lettuce. Plantain is an excellent cancer fighter because it cleanses the bloodstream. Chickweed and Dandelion are excellent for the blood and liver. Dandelion and Parsley are great for fluid retention. They are all blood builders because of the chlorophyll they contain. Blend all the greens well and strain and drink as much as you can in between meals. Don't drink with your meals as this slows down your digestion.

Don't eat any sugar products as pie, cake, ice cream, etc. Sugar in any form clogs our arteries and blood vessels. It destroys the white blood cells in our body which are the infection fighters. Sugar destroys the immune system in the process so you are susceptible to all kinds of disease from flu to cancer. Sugar leaches calcium out of the arteries and blood vessels weakening them. It takes calcium out of the bones, too. Sugar irritates the mucus membranes and causes fermentation in the body. Concentrated starches as pastas, noodles, spaghetti do the same thing as sugar because they turn to simple sugar in the body. Our pancreas can't handle all this simple sugar so it overworks and becomes weak as a result of trying to get the sugar out of the blood stream. Too much sugar in the blood stream leads to high blood pressure, diabetes, high cholesterol, strokes, and cancer to name a few.

Testimonials: This story is about 3 children born to one family. The first child a baby girl was born in 1951. She seemed perfectly normal at birth. However, after two months she became so pale her parents were very concerned. The doctor ordered a fast blood count, this revealed the fact that the baby had Leukemia. She was put in the hospital & within five and one-half days was given 25 blood transfusion. But all of this was fruitless & the baby girl died at the age of three months.

The second child a boy was born in 1953. The examination of the child's blood at birth revealed the terrifying fact that he, too, had Leukemia. The baby's doctor had become wise by now. He had become acquainted with the remarkable experience of Mrs. Catherine Ferraro, who had recovered from splenic Leukemia by taking large quantities of fresh raw carrot juice daily. The doctor was determined to save this boy. He called Mrs. Ferraro & asked her if she would bring fresh carrot juice to the hospital everyday. The Ferraros were not in the carrot juice business but they responded to the emergency. During the first three months of this baby's life all he drank was fresh made carrot juice. After three months his mother was told by the doctor to add fresh fruits & vegetables pureed in the blender. He ate no baby food out of a jar. He ate only fresh & raw foods. Did this juice therapy work? Much to the joy & amazement of all concerned at the end of one year the blood count was normal. There was no evidence of Leukemia. The carrot juice & raw foods had worked a miracle by making his diseased blood healthy. When he was five he was still doing well. He continues to drink his carrot juice everyday.

The third child a baby girl was born in 1954. A blood test at birth showed she had no Leukemia. What made the difference in the birth of these three children? Mother had been eating a terrible diet (the SAD American diet) of meat, dairy products, sweets, & etc. during the birth of the first two children. She became wiser when the third child was expected so she went on the mucusless diet of fruits, vegetables, whole grains, seeds, & nuts with a lot of fresh & raw, plus she drank carrot juice everyday. Just to be on the safe side this child was given nothing but carrot juice for the first three months of her life, too. At the age of four & five both were still drinking carrot juice everyday. They are the picture of health today.

The medical doctor treats Acute Leukemia very aggressively with chemotherapy which destroys the white blood cells. Now you have nothing to fight infection. Usually the infection in the lungs is what the patient succombs to not the Leukemia. The doctor doesn't allow you to have fresh fruits or vegetables which is what you need to replace the potassium that has leaked out of the cells. Remember chemotherapy destroys the immune system which is what you need to fight the Leukemia. The fresh & raw rebuild the immune system so the body can heal itself. Pray about it before you make a major decision.

God's Plan works if you treat it aggressively with 100% fresh & raw foods & raw vegetable juices with a natural healing doctor to monitor you.

DIGEST

Anyone with Cancer needs a digest aid with each meal as the undigested protein is feeding the Cancer so contact me for the Digest as it is the best.

Dr. Charles H. Andrus published his research report in the American Journal of Gastroenterology stating that the taking of an enzyme called cellulase is 83-100% effective in dissolving cellulose, which is the common component of bezoars. Even better news is if you take Digest with your meals you'll never have bezoars. All they are is undigested fiber which forms a mass in the stomach. This happens over a period of time because your foods are not being digested so the stomach doesn't pass it along to the next stage. Remember the entire digestive process works because of the presence of PLANT ENZYMES. None of the body processes can work without plant enzymes. Enzymes make energy production possible, they deliver nutrients to the cells and break down body fat. The white blood cells may become elevated when the food doesn't digest properly. ***DIGESTION PLAYS A PART IN ALL DISEASE***. Your organs require enzymes to function properly. Your body relies 100% on enzymes to fight off carcinogens, viruses, and bacteria. When you have cancer the body doesn't break down proteins and fats properly. The undigested proteins feed the cancer. The cancer cells feed on toxins and poisons in the system and the undigested protein is seen as a foreign body so it feeds the cancer cells and helps them grow. The enzymes help cancer by digesting the proteins so the immune system can destroy the cancer cells, too. Digest contains:

1. Cellulase-as stated earlier, it dissolves and prevents the accumulation of undigested foreign material in the stomach and small intestine. It digests the fiber in your foods.

2. Lipase-This is produced by the Pancreas if it is working properly. It is necessary for the digestion and absorption of fats. When you get older the amount of lipase produced by the body is dramatically reduced.

3. Maltase-this digests carbohydrates like maltose and starches. Researchers in the Neuroscience Center at the University of Tennessee have observed that a deficiency of maltase can cause respiratory failure.

4. Lactase-Low levels are responsible for lactose intolerance. Low levels can create abdominal discomfort. Antacids make this worse. Digest contains all the plant enzymes your body needs. Meat & dairy destroy the lactase.

5. Protease-This enzyme breaks down proteins so they can be digested. Scientists at the University of Massachusetts Medical Center have confirmed that the older we get the less able we are to digest & absorb the protein to maintain energy and muscle tone. Our body doesn't produce enough of the enzyme. Supplementation is the best way to get adequate amounts. Undigested protein floating around in the system causes excess mucus which causes bronchitis, flu, asthma, the undigested proteins cause Cancer & other diseases, etc.

6. Amylase-digests starches and carbohydrates.

You will find you do well if you have lots of the friendly bacteria. Digest contains 2 different kinds of the friendly bacteria in the colon to eat up the unfriendly bacteria such as ecoli or salmonella, or yeast infection, for example. THE UNFRIENDLY BACTERIA LIVE ON POISONS AND TOXINS. They love undigested foods. If you have bloating and cramping with pain in the stomach from undigested food, Digest will make this a thing of the past. This will put your digestive system's chemistry back in balance. It neutralizes and breaks down excess stomach acid. Rather than shutting down digestion entirely with acid-blocking drugs that upset the body's biochemical balance, enzymes keep the digestive process moving.

Proper food digestion is the key to maintaining your energy level and getting the proper absorption of nutrients from each meal. Enzyme deficiency is the problem with all disease. Indigestion, excess gas, burping, diarrhea, constipation, skin problems, bad breath, insomnia, nervousness, memory loss, mental fatigue are all as the result of poor digestion of your food. We need to have enzymes on a daily basis.

Any digest aid with animal enzymes will do you no good because they won't digest your food. One of them is pepsin. Don't take a digest aid with hydrochloric acid as this is telling the body it doesn't have to make it for digestion because here it comes. That is like a diabetic taking insulin. The Pancreas stops working because it is supplied by the shot of insulin. I recommend a well-balanced diet of fruits, vegetables, whole grains, seeds, and nuts. Follow an exercise program, too. If you eat all fresh and raw for a meal you may not need to take the enzymes as you will get enough enzymes in the 100% fresh fruit or raw vegetables.

Testimonial: One man had gas, bloating, and the gas pressed on the heart and caused pain so he thought he had heart trouble. He started on the digest aid with each meal. The result no gas, bloating, or pain. One happy man with no digestion problems.

I am enclosing some recipes since you are changing from a meat & dairy diet to all fruits, vegetables, whole grains, seeds, & nuts.

WHEAT-OAT CRACKERS

3/4 cup of whole wheat flour
3/4 cup quick oats
1/3 cup fine coconut or nut meal
1/4 cup plus 1 T. of warm water

Mix dry ingredients in a bowl. Add water all at once & mix well. Roll the dough out thinly & evenly to almost cover one regular cookie sheet. Dust the rolling pin with flour to prevent it from sticking to the dough. Score the crackers across the dough & up & down so you will have small pieces. Bake at 400 degrees for 15 minutes then at 250 until well dried out and lightly browned-watch it as it may not take long. Best fresh, but good later if stored in airtight container. Enjoy to your health.

CAROB PUDDING

1 cup of cold water   Bring 2 cups of water to a boil.
1/3 cup carob powder (Chatfield's)
2/3 cup sliced almonds
3 T. Raw honey
1 tsp. Vanilla
3 T. Cornstarch or arrowroot powder

Blenderize all in the left column until creamy (one minute). Bring the 2 cups of water to a boil and add the blended mixture to it, stirring constantly. When well thickened & creamy pour into pudding cups. Chill & serve.

ALMOND WHIPPED CREAM

2 & 3/4 CUP WATER
1 T. EACH (BARLEY FLOUR, CORNSTARCH, & RICE FLOUR)
2 T. RAW HONEY OR 6-8 PITTED DATES
1 CUP SLICED ALMONDS
1 & ½ TEASPOON VANILLA

BRING 2 CUPS OF WATER TO A BOIL, WHILE YOU BLENDERIZE THE OTHER INGREDIENTS IN THE REMAINING 3/4 CUP OF WATER. POUR BLENDED MIXTURE INTO THE BOILING WATER WHILE STIRRING CONSTANTLY. STIR COOK UNTIL THICKENED NICELY. COOL & SERVE AS YOU WOULD ANY WHIPPED CREAM. THE DIFFERENCE IS THIS ONE IS DAIRY FREE & PRESERVATIVE FREE.

MILLET PATTIES

2 cups of cooked millet (may add left over whole grain cereals to this)
½ cup of almond butter (I make my own) It is too thick so I add Barlean's flax oil to thin it some.
1 large chopped onion
Real Salt to season at the table
Add your favorite seasoning such as onion & garlic powder,

I use a T-fal pan, get it hot, form the patties-if too wet add cornmeal or flour so they form well. Put in the pan & fry until done on first side, turn & brown well. You may bake them at 350 degrees. Do not use any oil to fry or bake.

Cooking with the best oil like flax oil makes it harmful so it then is deposited on the arteries. These patties are delicious. Millet cereal is one of the best grains to eat as it is alkaline. This is one of my favorite patties. Serve on a whole wheat bun with eggless mayonnaise, alfalfa sprouts, tomatoes, onion, & loose-leaf lettuce. Enjoy to your heart's delight.

ALPINE CHEESE

½ cup of water
1/3 cup Emes unflavored gelatin
2 cups of hot cornmeal mush
1/3 cup-1/2 cup almond butter
1/4 cup lemon juice
1/4 cup yeast flakes
½ cup chopped onions
1/4 tsp. garlic powder
Add Realsalt to taste & blend well.

Cool the hot cornmeal mush, then whiz with the water & gelatin. Add the remaining ingredients & whiz thoroughly. This cheese is the best cheese for broiling, as it won't melt away as some of the homemade cheeses do. It is good on Pita bread as pizza or on your homemade pizza dough. You can get the can of green chili peppers for a hot cheese. I buy the can with the least amount of sodium. You can buy Barbara's unsalted blue corn chip at Kroger's in the health section or make your own crackers to eat with the cheese. Make sure you read labels & watch out they don't have canola or cottonseed oil in any chips or crackers you buy. I buy triscuits low sodium crackers. To make the cornmeal mush start with 2 cups of water, get it hot, then add ½ cup of cornmeal. Let it cook on low heat & stir with a wire whisk so it doesn't stick & clump together. You can dip chips in the cheese at first or let it thicken & slice it for sandwiches, etc.

Nut Milk

½ cup almonds-slivered
½ cup slivered almonds
1/8 cup or less honey
1 quart of water

Blend all until smooth. You may want to strain it. I save the fine particles to add to my whole grain cereal. You can use the nut milk as a base for homemade gravy.

ESSIAC FORMULA

Essiac is an herbal cancer remedy developed by Canadian nurse Rene Caisse(1888-1978). She has reportedly treated thousands of cancer patients through a period of 60 years, including many who were pronounced "hopeless" or "terminal" by orthodox doctors. The herbal tea formula was given to Rene by a hospital patient whose breast cancer was healed by an Ontario Indian. Caisse named the Indian formula Essiac (her name spelled backwards). She used it to treat cancer patients until the late 1970's.

Dr. Charles Brusch of the Brusch Medical Center, former physician to many members of the Massachusetts elite, including the late President John F. Kennedy, declared in 1959 that Essiac has merit in the treatment of cancer. Eight doctors petitioned the Canadian government in 1926 to let Caisse test the cancer remedy on a large scale. The doctors concluded that Essiac reduced tumor size, prolonged life, & showed "remarkably beneficial results" even in terminal cases where everything else has been tried without effect.

Rene Caisse's 72 year old mother was diagnosed as having inoperable liver cancer. Rene gave her mother daily injections of Essiac for months. Mrs. Caisse fully recovered from the cancer & lived to be 90. She died of heart disease with no cancer.

Caisse's hometown of Bracebridge, Ontario, Canada provided her with a hotel building for use as a cancer clinic. In 1937 Emma Carson, MD of Los Angeles, Calif. wrote a 5 page report on the clinic where she spent 245 days examining 400 patients. Dr. Carson wrote: The vast majority of Miss Caisse's patients were brought to her after surgery, radium, x-rays, etc had failed & the patients were pronounced incurable or hopeless cancer patients. The physicians sent the patients with letters certifying they had incurable or terminal cancer & had been given up by the medical profession as untreatable

The progress obtainable and the actual results from the Essiac treatments and the rapidity of repair were absolutely marvelous. Many patients listed as terminal without severe damage to life support organs were healed and lived 35-45 years or more with no cancer. Essiac is wonderful for stomach ulcers as they are gone in a month with daily use of the Essiac Formula.

Rene Caisse had clinical cases where a person on insulin discontinued it after taking Essiac. They concluded that the Essiac regulated the pancreas in cases of diabetes myelitis so these people became insulin free. Essiac gives you more energy & helps you to sleep like a baby as some "side effects". Study for yourself as there is so much more information about the product. Make sure you use a formula with all the herbs mentioned in this report. You can make it yourself or check with your local health food store to see if they have the formula with the 5 herbs. If they have a formula with only 4 herbs I would add the watercress to it myself.

The following is the directions for the Essiac Tea:

A four herb formula has oxalic acid in it because the hard tissue herbs need to be slow cooked not boiled to release the essential ingredients in some of the herbs. A five herb formula as given by Dr. Charles Brusch which should include the correct amount of water cress as this negates the effect of the oxalic acid. Remember, ill people often have weak kidneys to start with so this five formula is the best. The formula includes three hard tissue herbs (roots and bark) which are burdock, turkey rhubarb root, and slippery elm bark. The soft tissue herbs are sheep sorrel (leaves, stem, & flowers) & water cress.

THE HERBS SHOULD NEVER BE MIXED TOGETHER AND PLACED IN A POT & BOILED ALL TOGETHER UNLESS YOU PREMIX THE TURKEY RHUBARB, BURDOCK, & SLIPPERY ELM). They are the only ones that should be slow cooked. NEVER-NEVER SHOULD SOFT TISSUE HERBS BE BOILED. Heat kills the enzymes in these plants and it is the enzymes that your body uses to heal and repair itself. Enzymes start dying at 102 degrees F. and all are dead at 180 degrees F (boiling point is 212 F). The hard tissue herbs should be slow cooked to release the essential oils. The soft tissue herbs (sheep sorrel & water cress) need to be kept separate in a plastic bag so they are not heated with the other 3 herbs. It is best to take the herbs in a liquid or tea form as they go right to work. The liquid goes into the stomach & then right to the cells to begin the healing process.

1. Mix all the dry ingredients thoroughly (Place herbal contents in a large container with a lid & shake well. Remember to mix turkey rhubarb, burdock, & slippery elm only. Keep the watercress & sheep

sorrel leaves separate. I can order watercress powder for you. Use 2 ounces per 2 gallon of water.

2. Start with 2 gallons of the best water & bring to a rolling boil. Turn the burner down to simmer

3. Put 1 cup of three hard tissue herbs you have mixed (turkey rhubarb, burdock, & slippery elm) in the pot of water and continue slow cooking for 10 minutes.

4. Turn off the burner, scrape down the sides & stir the mixture thoroughly, put a lid on the pan.

5. Allow the herbs in the pot to steep for 12 hours (keep the lid closed) then turn the burner on & heat on simmer about 20 minutes. This finishes steeping out the active herbal ingredients. Don't let the mixture boil as this destroys the essential oils. Turn off the burner. Add 1 cup of the soft tissue herbs (sheep sorrel & water cress). Let these steep in the other mixture for 4 hours with a lid on the pan. Strain the herbs out of the mixture. Run through a strainer and then through a cotton cloth.

Dry Ingredients-Herbs

24 oz. Burdock Root
16 oz. Sheep Sorrel-Powdered or leaves
1 oz. Turkey Rhubarb Root-Powdered
4 oz. Slippery Elm Bark-Powdered
6 ozs. of fresh water cress or 2 ozs. powdered water cress.

Keep the 2 combinations of herbs in a sealed plastic bag for future use.

Sterilize your bottles and pour the cool strained tea in the bottles. Tighten the bottles after it has cooled sufficiently. Store in a cool place or in the refrigerator as there are no preservatives in it. If mold should develop discard immediately. You can add some lemon juice to each bottle as a natural preservative. Shake the bottle before each use. Take 2 ozs. of it twice a day. In the morning upon arising, one hour or more before eating is best. Take at bedtime on an empty stomach or at least 2 hours after eating. In severe cases take 2 oz. before noon meal, also.

Note: If you have severe stomach problems, mix 1 T. of powdered Slippery Elm with 2 cups of water, shake well or put in the blender to mix & drink a few ounces before taking the Essiac Formula. The Slippery Elm heals any raw irritated areas as ulcers or acid reflux, etc. Do not microwave it as this destroys it.

Locally grown organic herbs are superior to imported herbs. Be careful in your herb purchases. Many herbs are imported, non-medicinal grade and not harvested properly. Ask about the herbs before you buy them.

You need to do a good health program. Eat only fresh fruits, vegetables, whole grains, seeds, & nuts. Meat & dairy products feeds the cancer because the Cancer cells have a protein coating on them to protect themselves. They love undigested protein & they get plenty if you are not taking a digest aid. Read about Digest in my Cancer book. Your body isn't breaking down the proteins & fats properly. Follow the whole program in my Cancer book as there is not one magic answer for Cancer. My Cancer book would be a good investment as it gives you a full program to follow so the body can heal itself through a strong immune system.

Proverbs 17:22 It reads "A merry heart doeth good like a medicine."

Proverbs 26:2 "The curse causeless shall not come".

Remember we are what we eat. Gen.1:29 is God's diet for us.

Miracle 2 Products

We are distributors for some 100% natural products that you can take internally as they will alkalinize the system while they detoxify. This allows the body to heal itself. You can take the neutralizer internally either the liquid or the gel. This is good for all types of health problems from colds to cancer. When you take it internally it goes right to the cells to neutralize any problem. If you have a headache take some of the neutralizer to alkalinize & detoxify the system. Soon you have no headache. Listen to your body. Start with 10 drops and add more as you need it. Put the neutralizer in water. Remember it detoxifies while it alkalinizes the system getting rid of the acidity. You can replace every chemical in your home. There are many ways to use the soap & the neutralizer. You can pull out toxins while soaking in the tub with hot water, some soap & at least one ounce of the Neutralizer. Soak for at least 45 minutes to one hour for aches & pains. Save the bath water to water your plants as they will grow superbly because they have all the nutrients they need. Use one ounce of neutralizer & one ounce of the soap/gallon of water for bugs on plants. Spray the fruit trees & water the roots good with the bath water to feed the plants. They are getting all the nutrients they need for healthy growth. Spray the neutralizer on your rose bushes after they leaf out & you will have beautiful roses. Use 2 oz. of the Neutralizer/gallon of water. In New England they raise cranberries. Moths were coming that destroy the crop. They put the soap & neutralizer in the sprinkling system & left the sprinklers on for one minute directing it to the moths & all the moths were destroyed. Blueberry farmers put the neutralizer & soap in the irrigation system & got wonderful berries.

The Neutralizer gel is 3 times stronger than the neutralizer & it is a concentrate. You can take it for heartburn or acid reflux a teaspoon or a T. at a time. It is soothing to the stomach, also. When you have Acid Reflux the digestion is very poor. You need A digest aid like Digest. Don't eat a heavy meal at night eat fruit & toast or homemade soup & toast & you will do better, also, with the Acid Reflux at night. Keep the gel by the bed.

Testimonial: A medical doctor is using it with his patients. He tells them to take one ounce of Neutralizer in a quart of water with one drop of the Miracle 2 soap & many are passing parasites. One man passed a 15 foot tape worm.

Testimonial: A lady has a 10 year old grandson with 10-15 warts on the bottom of his feet & they are very painful. The mother started rubbing the Neutralizer on them & the warts were gone in over a month. He has MS & he is taking baths with the soap & 1 ounce of the Neutralizer. She rubs him after the bath with the Neutralizer & it is helping him besides taking it internally.

Testimonials: One man had an infection in his eye. He was on antibiotics for it but it just got worse. The doctor said he would have to remove his eyeball so it wouldn't spread. He heard about the Miracle 2 products & he took an oz. of the Neutralizer internally & began washing his eyes with the neutralizer & putting drops of it in the eyes. He put the Neutralizer gel in his eyes & now the infection is all gone. He saved his eyesight with the Neutralizer. It helps pyorrhea & gum problems, also. You can brush your teeth with one or 2 drops of the soap & the teeth get white & the plaque just falls off. Your mouth will foam with the soap on the brush but remember it is 100% natural you can swallow it & get rid of parasites. A lady went to the dentist for her 6 months cleaning.

The dental hygienist said your teeth are clean. She asked, "What do you mean?" She said your teeth are polished & they don't need any more cleaning. There was no plaque. She was happy. She was using the soap & the gel for some time on her teeth.

Testimonial: A man had glaucoma that the pressure was building up more each time he was examined by the eye doctor. The doctor wanted to put him on a drug that he would be on for the rest of his life. He refused & started on the Neutralizer & gel washing his eyes with the liquid & putting the gel & liquid in his eyes. In 2 weeks the pressure was normalized. He took an ounce of the Neutralizer internally to clean the toxins out so he would have better circulation to the eyes. His glaucoma got better & better.

Testimonial: A man smoked a pipe all his adult life. He had emphysema so bad he couldn't drive a car & had no energy to do anything. He doesn't smoke any more. He started to put the neutralizer in his nebulizer & was taking many ounces of the neutralizer internally everyday. He does his soaks 3 times a week. He now has more energy, is breathing better, now drives his car & is more independent. You can write your own testimonial of what it has done for you.

Soak in the tub with one oz. of the Neutralizer & some of the soap & it will pull out toxins & take away aches & pains. You can put the gel on your knees for arthritis, weak cartilage or for any ache you have rub it into the area well. Put the gel on for scrapes, cuts, & burns as it heals. Take the gel internally for heartburn & much more. After you soak in the tub apply the gel & then run the laundry ball over the sore spots.

Testimonial: 86 year old lady needed 5 way bypass. The lady consulted with her sons & she decided to "pass on" the 5-way by-pass surgery. She began an intense Miracle 2 program. She soaked in the tub one hour, with a capful of soap & one capful of the Neutralizer. Then she put a lot of the Gel over the heart area on the chest, followed by an absorbent pad wet with the Neutralizer. She used hospital type bed pads, cut to size, as they already had one side plastic & one side absorbent. She took the neutralizer internally & in a few months she went in for more tests & the doctors found no reason for by-pass surgery this time.

Testimonial: A lady had lung & liver Cancer. She was given 6 months to live by her medical doctor (who made him God)? She changed her diet & chose God's diet of fruits, vegetables, whole grains, seeds, & nuts. She prayed that God would show her what to do as she didn't want to die. The next day a package came from her uncle with the Miracle 2 soap & neutralizer. There was a note with it telling her how to use the products. She soaked in the tub with one ounce of the soap & one ounce of the Neutralizer for one hour & the water was very murky dark brown in color. The soap & neutralizer in the water opened up her billions of pores & drew out poisons thru her skin. She was excited & she kept doing the baths 3 times a week. She took the neutralizer internally & took some of the gel as well. She put her trust in the Lord & prayed for total healing while she was doing the Miracle 2 program & eating God's diet. She studied her Bible & asked other people to remember her in prayer & in 6 months she was well. She tells everyone about the Miracle 2 products & what they did for her.

A Massage Therapist tells us the following testimonials: After a long day of working outside I was left with three blisters on my thumb and first finger. I was afraid to pop them for fear of infection, but also knew I couldn't work with them that way. I plastered them with the Miracle2 Gel & Neutralizer and went to bed. The next morning there was no sign of the blisters!!! That's a miracle!!! Many of my clients have benefitted from the Miracle products too. One client had painful shingles. I let her use some of the Skin moisturizer and overnight her shingles stopped itching or hurting, and dried up, and haven't come back.

Alkaline, Ionized Water

After 65 years of research & testing the Japanese determined that the 3 major causes of old age, sickness, & disease are free radicals, dehydration & acidosis.

Our bodies are 80% water so in order to be free of disease you want the best water. You need to drink restructured alkaline water.

Our brain is 90% water, when it can't maintain that % it pulls water from other parts of the body. Reverse osmosis & distilled water are dead water & they leach minerals out of the body & dehydrate the body.

Alkaline ionized water electrolysis converts the inorganic minerals in the water to organic minerals just like plant juice. When the water goes through the machine the process pulls all the acidic minerals such as fluoride, chlorine, arsenic, lead, etc & restructures them by the electrolysis process out of 1 hose & leaves only the alkaline minerals for drinking with organic calcium, magnesium, & potassium coming through another hose. Alkaline, ionized water is the most powerful liquid antioxidant that can help rebuild the immune system & it is revolutionizing the health industry. It allows greater penetration into the cells than any other water & it reduces wrinkles because the skin is also getting the water it needs. It hydrates the whole body & cleanses the acid out on a daily basis.

When the body is too acidic it builds fat cells to protect itself from the acidity. Most people with diabetes, for example, are overweight. When an overweight person drinks the alkaline, ionized water faithfully they lose inches in a few months. They look better & feel better. An increase in consumption of the alkaline water reduces the fat deposits so you lose weight naturally. Drink 50% of your body's weight in ounces of alkaline water.

The kidneys can't function properly without enough water so some of the load is dumped onto the liver. One of the liver's many functions is to metabolize stored fat into usable energy. If the liver has to do some of the kidney's work it can't do what it should.

The alkalizer is a commercial machine made for home use. It is manufactured by a family company in Japan. One in 5 homes in Japan have a water machine. They are registered as a Medical device in Japan & used in hospitals with wonderful results.

You can cook with it & your vegetables get done sooner. It attaches to your faucet at your kitchen sink. The main hose gives you good tasting alkaline water & a smaller hose gives you acidic water. The acidic water kills ecoli & salmonella & other contaminants so you can wash your fruits & vegetables in it. In Japan in their restaurants they wash their counter tops with only the acidic water & they are free of germs. The acidic water on the skin heals eczema, dermatitis, cysts, burns, & much more.

David Baltes, the President of the Alkalizer Company visited every manufacturing plant in Japan that makes water machines looking for the best machines 13 years ago. They have a 5 year warranty on the machine. David has lots of testimonials to share.

Go to alkalizer.com & listen to the video by David Baltes & you will get excited. We explored the water industry for 5 months looking for the best & the most economical & affordable machine that does what it says. We feel like the Lord led us to the alkalizer. I talked to David Baltes several times.

Call Dawn to order your machine. You can become a distributor if you want & share it with other people or just buy one for your family & share the water with friends. Their hours are 11 AM to 5 PM (EST). Her phone is 407-226-3701 tell her Joyce Trout referred you & leave your phone # & she'll call you back. Let me know if you have any questions about the machine. My phone number is 931-498-2844.

Joyce gave a lecture every day for 5 days at a medical missionary school several years ago & we have put the lectures on 5 DVD's. You can have the set of 5 for the incredible price of only $85. There is one hour to an hour & 20 minutes of herbal talks on each DVD giving you herbal formulas for different health challenges, plus healthful information for general well being.

You will find what to do for different diseases such as asthma, gangrene, bleeding of the lungs, bedsores, bronchitis, ulcers, lung problems, pyorrhea, varicose veins, & much more. God's Plan works if we work the Plan. Joyce has written a book on Cancer, Diabetes, Strokes, & a Vegan Cookbook & she is looking for Medical Missionaries to sell her books for God's ailing people. You would buy them at wholesale & sell them for retail. Call Joyce at 931-498-2844

www.ingramcontent.com/pod-product-compliance
Lightning Source LLC
Chambersburg PA
CBHW022103170526
45157CB00004B/1457